AF553583

Manual of
Reconstructive Hand Surgery

G Karthikeyan MBBS MS MCh (Plastic Surgery)
Assistant Professor
Institute for Research and Rehabilitation of Hand and
Department of Plastic Surgery
Stanley Medical College and
Government Hospital
Chennai, Tamil Nadu, India

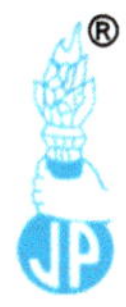

JAYPEE BROTHERS MEDICAL PUBLISHERS (P) LTD

New Delhi • London • Philadelphia • Panama

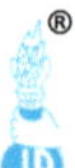

Jaypee Brothers Medical Publishers (P) Ltd.

Headquarters
Jaypee Brothers Medical Publishers (P) Ltd.
4838/24, Ansari Road, Daryaganj
New Delhi 110 002, India
Phone: +91-11-43574357
Fax: +91-11-43574314
Email: jaypee@jaypeebrothers.com

Overseas Offices

J.P. Medical Ltd.
83, Victoria Street, London
SW1H 0HW (UK)
Phone: +44-2031708910
Fax: +02-03-0086180
Email: info@jpmedpub.com

Jaypee-Highlights Medical Publishers Inc.
City of Knowledge, Bld. 237, Clayton
Panama City, Panama
Phone: +507-301-0496
Fax: +507-301-0499
Email: cservice@jphmedical.com

Jaypee Brothers Medical Publishers Ltd.
The Bourse
111, South Independence Mall East
Suite 835, Philadelphia, PA 19106, USA
Phone: +267-519-9789
Email: joe.rusko@jaypeebrothers.com

Jaypee Brothers Medical Publishers (P) Ltd.
17/1-B, Babar Road, Block-B, Shaymali
Mohammadpur, Dhaka-1207
Bangladesh
Mobile: +08801912003485
Email: jaypeedhaka@gmail.com

Jaypee Brothers Medical Publishers (P) Ltd.
Shorakhute, Kathmandu
Nepal
Phone: +00977-9841528578
Email: jaypee.nepal@gmail.com

Website: www.jaypeebrothers.com
Website: www.jaypeedigital.com

Inquiries for bulk sales may be solicited at: jaypee@jaypeebrothers.com

Manual of Reconstructive Hand Surgery

First Edition: 2013, Reprint: **2024**
ISBN: 978-93-5090-512-8
Printed in India

Dedicated to

My Gurus and patients

Preface

Hand surgery is more an art form. This is because we are dealing with living, moving and gliding delicate tissues that respond positively to gentle dissection and react violently to unsure steps, rough handling and disregard for hemostasis. I remember reading somewhere that a hand surgeon must be in and out of the tissues before the tissues are even aware of the intrusion. This, I suppose, was said, because the lesser the tissue handling, the better will be the results, as the postoperative inflammation and edema will be minimal. To achieve this, speed is of prime importance, and must be accompanied by gentle tissue handling.

Such tissue handling can be minimized if the surgeon is aware of what to do, how to do and when to do. Avoiding unnecessary steps, circumventing potential problems in dissection, undoing mistakes, and taking extra care at strategic points are some of the ways in which a smooth conduct of the surgical procedure can be achieved.

At the beginning of my career in hand surgery, I was lucky to be guided by experts in the field, as they led me step by step through the many procedures. However, elaborate textbooks may be on the descriptive aspects of the surgical procedures, but they may not suffice for a beginner who is attempting for the first time, even a well-described procedure.

So, I envisaged *Manual of Reconstructive Hand Surgery*, which will play the role of a coach and also be able to guide the surgeon throughout the procedure. This book is written with this intention.

I hope, this book will help surgeons to carry out their procedures with ease. After all, the ultimate beneficiary should be the patient.

The procedures have been described in practical and easy way, and may not be the original description.

G Karthikeyan

Contents

Section 1 • General Considerations

Section 2 • Skin Reconstruction

Introduction

When the patient presents in the outpatient room and seeks consultation, he is harboring a lot of hopes and aspirations; expects his hand to get back to normal after treatment.

It is the bounden duty of the hand surgeon to fulfill the expectations of the patient as far as possible. At the same time, the practical outcomes should be explained to the patient.

The diagnosis is obvious. For example, the diagnosis of brachial plexus injury may be made quite easily within a minute of meeting the patient. Similarly, conditions, such as post burn contractures can be diagnosed even by just looking at the patient. So, it is not the diagnosing that is required or important in the hand surgery. What is required is the workup of the patient that will lead surgeons to make a plan for management. This plan should take into account a lot of factors, such as sex of the patient, occupation, side involved, and even the age of the patient. This book is compiled with these aims.

This is not a textbook, but a practical guide for the nascent hand surgeons. The book will help the hand surgeons to conduct a rehearsal in the mind the day before the surgery.

In making assessment of hand-injured patients, a lot depends on the type of tissue injured, such as skin, bone or tendon. So, the main part of the book is devoted to the management of such conditions involving the different tissues in different sections.

This book contains 18 sections. Each section has three segments:

1. The first segment is on assessment of the problem, so that a correct understanding of the situation can be made. Based on this, the decision can be made about the management protocol.
2. The second segment deals with presenting a simplified management protocol, which will be deduced from the needs of the patient and the findings made on assessment of the problem in the previous segment. It will not give all the options, but the one that is most useful and what is routinely used.
3. The third segment describes the main surgical procedures enumerated in the management protocol. Just reading through this segment will not be enough qualification to perform the procedure. The surgeon must know the technique by reading about it first from a standard textbook, then watching, and then assisting at the surgical procedures being performed by a qualified surgeon. When the surgical procedure is being done, this manual will help:
   - By giving a simplified description of the steps of the surgery
   - By listing out the steps and thus avoiding missed steps
   - By giving useful tips at various steps
   - By suggesting troubleshooting measures in cases of probable difficulties
   - By giving warning about difficult steps.

The section 15 deals with common hand conditions faced by the hand surgeons and also pose problems in both assessment and planning. Examples are brachial plexus injuries and Volkmann's ischemic contractures. Such conditions are also dealt with in three segments.
At the end, there are two useful sections: Appendices and Proformas.

The section on appendices gives instructions on useful day-to-day procedures. Starting from how to prepare for the hand surgery and how to set up the infrastructure before a microsurgical procedure. This section also gives a list of instruments and equipment required in an operation theater to start the hand surgery and microsurgery. These are used in various hand surgery procedures, and include harvesting skin grafts, nerve grafts, etc.

The section on proformas gives many forms that can be used in the outpatient block when the patient is being examined. These forms are based on the assessment parameters of the individual conditions and ensure that all the parameters are assessed without missing any detail. They may also serve as databases containing all the relevant details that can be used in any retrospective study.

So, this is a cook book!

- Starting from the patient entering the outpatient block—practical steps to deal with the situations
- How to diagnose
- How to decide what to do
- How to decide time for doing procedure
- Preoperative counseling
- How to prepare for the procedure

} in the section Assessment

- How to do the procedure
- How to follow-up the patient

} in the section on Procedure

Knowing all the procedures described here will *not make a complete hand surgeon. He/she must know all the other procedures and the methods of doing them.*

SECTION

1

General Considerations

Examination of the Hand

1

When the patient presents in the outpatient clinic, there is a set protocol to be followed.

Seating the Patient

- If the patient is an adult, he is first asked to be seated comfortably, preferably on the right side of the examiner. This position is more comfortable for conducting the examination.
- If the patient is a child, the child can be more comfortably examined if he is on his mother's or grandmother's lap.
- If the patient is an infant, he can be made to lie on the examination couch with adequate protective pillows on either side. If the baby is fidgety, he can be held by his mother or grandparent on the shoulder and the child's hands can be examined from behind. The complete examination of the baby may not be possible in one consultation, especially in cases like birth palsy. This is because, this condition will show changes with time, and these changes should be tracked religiously. It will require serial consultations before a definite diagnosis and plan of management may be made.

Communicating with the Patient

- Developing a rapport with the patient is a very important part of the initial examination. Hand surgery is a specialty where the patient-doctor relationship is significant for many reasons:
- Deciding the management depends on multivarious factors ranging from the age, occupation, needs of the patient and sometimes even what the patient wants. The surgeon can get a clear idea about the patient only if the patient is able to communicate freely and without fear or apprehension.
- Many of the procedures require a long follow-up period. Only if the patient is able to communicate with the surgeon and vice-versa, this may be possible.
- Some of the surgical procedures require multiple stages and the entire reconstruction may take several months. It is important that the patient trusts the surgeon and attends each surgical stage.
- Some of the procedures like micro-surgical toe transfers require the transfer of one normal part of the body to another part which has been lost. Hence, there exists a small risk of failure and the consequence is that the patient loses another part of his body due to the surgical procedure. It is the responsibility of the surgeon to talk to the patient about this and it is also important for the patient to have trust in the surgeon if he agrees for the procedure.
- Some procedures like neurotization procedures for brachial plexus injury may have a long period before any

change can be manifest. This should be informed to the patient and the patient will be able to understand this only if the bond with the surgeon is strong.
- Legible language should be used when communicating with the patient. It is ideal that the conversation takes place in the patient's native language. This is because the patient must be able to understand correctly what is required of him. When the hand is being tested for specific movements and the action of specific muscles, surgeon should give clear instructions as to how the movement should be done, and if necessary, demonstrate it on his own hand, before the patient is asked to do it.
- If the patient is a child, the pros and cons of the treatment options must be discussed with the parents of the child if possible, or the guardians of the child.

Eliciting the History

As in any medical examination, the history plays an important role. In patients with hand injury, there are a few points to be emphasized while eliciting the history. The general points are discussed here, but there are specific details required in different conditions which will be dealt with in the relevant sections.
- Nature of complaints
- Duration of complaints
- Exact date of injury if any
- History of previous treatment

Examination of the Patient

This book has described in detail, the examination of the different tissues of the hand, such as skin, bone, tendon, nerve, etc. So it is mandatory that a preliminary diagnosis be made of the tissue involved before the appropriate examination is conducted. Sometimes, the involvement is not restricted to one tissue alone like tendon or bone. It may encompass different tissues and all these should be identified in the preliminary examination. There are a few pointers which will help surgeon to identify the problem.

Then the assessment of the problem is made as described in the appropriate chapter:
- If there is a raw area → go to chapter on *raw areas on skin*
- If there is evidence of adherent skin or scar → go to chapter on *other problems of skin*
- If there are no movements in parts of the hand or movements of the finger are not full → go to chapter on *tendons* and *nerves* to identify the problem
- If movements lost and sensation lost → go to chapter on *nerves*
- If there is a deformity of bone, or abnormal mobility is present in the area of bone → go to chapter on *bone assessment*
- If there is no movement at a joint → go to chapter on *joints*
- If there is a postburn contracture → go to chapter on *contractures*
- If there is a paralysis/weakness of the hand alone → go to chapter on *Hansens*
- If there is a history of injury in the neck or shoulder area, and there is some loss of movements in the upper limb → go to the section on *traumatic brachial plexus injuries*
- If there is a history of no movements of the upper limb noticed immediately after birth → go to the chapter on *obstetric brachial plexus injuries* to help in evaluation and management.
- If there is evidence of involvement of multiple tissues like skin and tendon, or tendon and bone, the sequence of management is described in the chapter on *complex post-traumatic problems.*
- If there is a problem of the thumb, it is dealt with in the chapter on *thumb reconstruction.*

And, based on the assessment, the plan of surgery can be made. This is also described in the same chapter as the assessment.

No clinical diagnosis is complete without making a plan of the sequence of management. There are many modalities of management, like physiotherapy, splints, and surgical procedures either in multiple stages or in a single stage. A logical sequence of management should be made which should suit the needs of the patient, and which will result in a useful function on the involved hand.

SECTION

2

Skin Reconstruction

Assessment of Skin Loss on the Hand

2

Introduction

This chapter refers to skin loss and raw areas that are not seen in the emergency situation, but at a time that is beyond the stage of primary reconstruction.

Resurfacing an area of skin loss is a common problem for a hand surgeon. The causes leading to skin loss on the hands are very much, the most common being trauma. Other causes include burns including electrical burns and infections. There are other situations like tumors, burn contractures and congenital anomalies where skin loss becomes apparent after the condition is operated on. Such conditions will be dealt with later. This chapter deals with apparent raw areas that need skin cover.

Before planning for treatment of a raw area on the hand, a systematic assessment is required. Only a correct evaluation of the problem can lead to a suitable surgical option being chosen as management. Achieving a good skin cover on the hand is not the goal, but achieving good function in the hand is the ultimate aim. All our efforts in choosing a skin cover must be focused on the issue of achieving function.

Qualities of an ideal skin cover for a defect on the hand:

- Must be durable skin
- Must be cosmetically pleasing
- Must be sensate
- Must be pain-free.

The surgical procedure that is planned for the patient ideally:

- Must be a single-staged procedure
- Must have minimal or no donor site morbidity
- Must have only a negligible risk factor
- Should be easy to perform.

Assessment of the Raw Area

Site of the defect: The exact location of the defect must be noted. Defects in different areas require different types of skin cover. A defect on the pulp of the thumb requires a skin cover that is sensate to allow the thumb to function normally. However, there are certain flaps that are designed for typical defects. Raw areas on the volar aspect of the fingers can be covered with cross-finger flaps from the adjoining finger.

Size of the defect: The size of the defect is important for planning a skin cover. Small defects may be covered with local flaps. If, however, the defect is larger, other flaps may have to be thought of.

Shape of the defect: The direction and shape of the defect can also influence the plan.

Floor of the defect: If the floor of the defect exposes bone or tendon, a vascularized skin cover is required.

Edges of the defect: The edges of the defect are important in deciding on the plan of skin cover. If the edges are unhealthy or macerated, the skin cover planned should be larger than the actual defect itself as the debridement of unhealthy tissues is of paramount importance. If the edges are everted or rolled out, suggesting a malignancy, the total plan may be different.

Distal deficit: A careful assessment of the distal finger or hand must be made.

1. *Associated tendon injury or loss:* If there is an associated injury or loss of tendon; either flexor or extensor, the skin flap should be given first and the tendon reconstruction can be done later when the skin flap has settled and become soft and supple. Simultaneous reconstruction of the tendons also along with the skin cover is done only in situations where the skin flap that has been planned is a free flap like the anterolateral thigh flap where 100 percent inset is given, i.e. the flap completely covers the defect and no area is exposed to the environment. Simultaneous reconstruction of the tendons can also be done if a pedicled island flap like the radial artery forearm flap or a posterior interosseous artery flap is used for skin cover as these flaps also provide total inset.
2. *Associated bone fracture with or without loss:* Skeletal stability is essential before planning a skin cover. However, if there is a fracture, internal fixation through a raw area is not prescribed. But stability must be achieved and this can be done by the use of external fixators that can stabilize the skeleton when the skin cover is given. When there is a bone loss, primary bone grafting is not advised and must be done at a later date after the skin reconstruction is

Table 2.2.1 Assessment of raw area and surgical plan

Site of raw area	*Characteristic*	*Surgical plan*
Single finger	Defect on volar aspect alone	Cross-finger flap (CFF)
	Defect on dorsal aspect alone	Reverse dorsal cross-finger flap (RDCFF)
	Defect on dorsum of PPX alone	Reverse dorsal metacarpal artery flap
Multiple fingers	Defect on volar aspect alone	Abdominal flap-superiorly based
	Defect on dorsal aspect alone	Abdominal flap-inferiorly based
Thumb	Skin loss on the pulp	Neurovascular island flap of littler
	Skin loss on the dorsum up to the interphalangeal (IP) joint	First dorsal metacarpal artery flap
Loss of thumb or circumferential loss on the fingers		Groin flap
Skin loss on the dorsum of hand	With less expertise	Abdominal flap-inferiorly based
	With more expertise	Posterior interosseous artery flap
Skin loss on the palm	With less expertise	Abdominal flap-superiorly based
	With more expertise	Reverse flow radial artery flap
End-on defect	On the thumb	Staged island flap of Professor R Venkataswami
	On multiple fingers	End-on groin flap
Large defects on the hand	With less expertise	Quadrant flap
	With microsurgical expertise	Free anterolateral thigh flap
Degloving injury of the entire hand and fingers		Buried abdominal flap

over. In the meantime, to achieve stability, external fixators can be applied. Primary reconstruction of the skin and bone can be done if a free flap or pedicled island flap is planned as skin cover.

3. *Associated nerve injury or loss:* This should be reconstructed after the skin reconstruction is over unless a free or pedicled island flap is used as skin cover.

Table 2.2.1 shows the assessment of raw area and surgical planning.

> The commonly used flaps like the cross finger flap, abdominal flap and groin flap are not discussed in this manual.

Assessment of the Patient

Certain points are to be remembered when deciding on skin cover:

- *Very anxious patients:* Select a safe and time-tested flap. Leave very little margin for failure or complications.
- *Mentally unsound patients:* Select a single-staged flap. Choosing a staged flap like the groin or abdominal flap may result in complications as the patient will not be compliant.
- *Children:* Usually are very compliant for even pedicled flaps like groin or abdominal flaps.
- *Elderly patients:* Avoid staged procedures. These may cause stiffness of joints. Select the simplest procedure.

Always talk to the patient about the procedure, the postoperative period and possible outcome. Get their full consent before embarking on the surgery. Even if the patient is a child of school going age, talk with him. Their level of understanding will sometimes surprise surgeon!

Littler's Island Flap

3

Introduction

The flap of choice for the reconstruction of a defect on the pulp region of the thumb is a neurovascular island flap described by Littler.

Advantages

- It brings partly glabrous skin to the pulp of thumb which is well padded, durable and cosmetically appealing.
- It is sensate and hence the function of the thumb is not interfered with.
- It is a single staged procedure.

Disadvantages

- It requires a surgical expertise in performing this procedure.
- It entails significant donor site morbidity—there is loss of sensation on the ulnar half of the middle finger, there is a significant scarring on the middle finger.
- Sensory re-education is necessary to get appreciable sensation on the flap.

Presurgical Counseling

- This procedure is planned to cover the raw area on the thumb with skin and tissues with sensation.
- This procedure will be done under axillary block anesthesia or GA in children.
- This procedure will take about 3 hours to perform.
- Skin will be removed along with soft tissues from the middle finger and placed on the raw area of the thumb. This will entail making incisions on the palm also. A skin graft will be taken from the medial side of the upper arm and applied over the secondary raw area on the middle finger. There will be a loss of sensation on one side of the middle finger and there will be a scar on the finger. There will also be a scar on the medial side of the arm.
- Admission will be necessary for a minimum period of 3 days
- A dressing will be applied and a plaster of Paris (POP) will be applied, which will be retained for 10 days, following which, physiotherapy will be started. At the beginning, when the thumb is touched, it will feel as if the middle finger is being touched. During the period of physiotherapy, techniques will be taught to make the sensation more natural. The sensation that returns may not be equal to the sensation on the normal thumb.
- A splint will have to be applied on the ring finger for a period of 3 to 4 weeks afterward.
- In some instances, the flap may not be possible because of anatomical variations. In such cases, other surgery like a cross-finger flap may be done.

- The general complications of local anesthetic infiltration like hypersensitivity may occur in spite of test dose application. This complication will cause dryness of mouth and apprehension, which can be corrected immediately.

Surgical Steps

1. The preferred anesthesia is either axillary block or general anesthesia (in children).
2. Apply the tourniquet and keep ready.
3. Preparation and draping as described in Appendix I.
4. The elbow area must also be prepared and kept exposed.
5. Raise the tourniquet and note the time.
6. Debride the defect and measure it. Make sure that the edges consist of intact and healthy skin. Take a lint pattern of the defect.

> Take the marking of the flap about 0.25 cm more on all sides as this is a thick flap and may be too tight if measurements are taken exactly.

7. Markings for the flap:
   - Draw a line from the ulnar border of the radially abducted thumb extending into the palm. Draw another longitudinal line from the web between middle and ring fingers proximally into the palm. The point at which these two lines intersect is point "A", the pivot point of the flap
   - Place the lint piece of the defect over the defect and cut a lint pedicle up to point "A" (Fig. 2.3.1).
   - Holding the lint at point "A", transpose the lint of the defect to the middle finger on the ulnar side. It should not go beyond the distal interphalangeal (DIP) crease of the middle finger
   - The flap can now be marked on the middle finger ulnar side keeping in mind the following criteria: the flap should not go beyond the mid volar line or the mid dorsal line (Fig. 2.3.2). Distally, surgeon should remember that the nail bed extends for 3 to 4 mm proximal to the nail fold, hence the flap should not go beyond this area

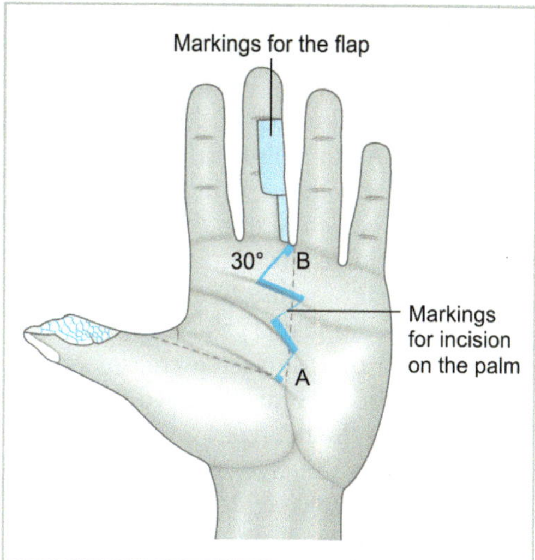

Fig. 2.3.1 Markings for the flap

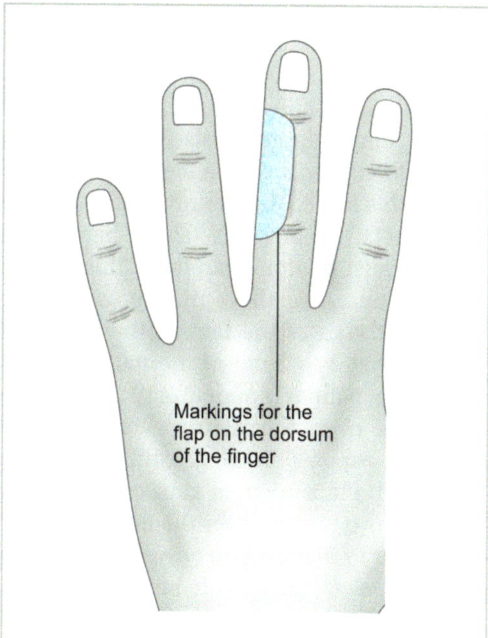

Fig. 2.3.2 Markings on the dorsum of finger

- From the proximal border of the flap, make a marking on the ulnar neutral line till the web area to reach point "B".
- Now draw the axis of the flap, i.e. from point "A" to point "B". However, this should not be a straight incision, as it will lead to a straight line scar that may lead to a contracture. It should be a zigzag line marked with two considerations: (1) the axis of the flap and (2) the transverse creases on the palm. From point "B", move at an angle of 30° to the nearest transverse crease, run along the crease till you cross the axis line. Now, again move to the next proximal transverse crease and when you reach it, run along the crease till you cross the axis line. Then move directly to point "A". This is the marking for the incision.

8. First make the incisions marked from "A" to "B". This incision should go through the skin and the subcutaneous tissue, till the palmar aponeurosis is seen. Lift up this thick fascia with a forceps and open it with a knife. The neurovascular bundle is directly below this fascia, hence this step must be done carefully. This should be done along the entire length of the marked axis of the flap. Remember that the distal 2 to 3 cm of the palm will not have a palmar aponeurosis. When this step is over, the neurovascular bundle will be exposed in the proximal 2/3 of the wound. Place a small gauze soaked in 1 percent xylocaine over the neurovascular bundle to prevent the vessels from going into spasm. There will be about 4 to 6 triangular flaps that must be raised and anchored with 3.0 ethilon to enhance the exposure and facilitate further dissection.
9. The dissection of the vascular pedicle begins here. Gently hold the soft tissues around the neurovascular bundle with a Jeweler's forceps and examine the anatomy. One digital nerve and one digital artery will be seen. The digital nerve will be seen to divide into two branches to supply the middle and ring fingers. Gently tease the tissues between the two branches of the common digital nerve and keep separating them proximally. Never dissect between the digital artery and the nerves. Dissect only to separate the ring finger digital nerve away from the bundle. Again it is reiterated that dissection should never be done between the digital artery and the digital nerve to the middle finger as it damages the minute veins that serve as venous drainage for the flap. Stop when the digital nerve of the ring finger has been separated up to the pivot point. Now cauterize gently the small branches from the digital artery to the deeper tissues. Now the neurovascular bundle has been dissected free in the palm. The pad of fat in the web space must be carefully teased to expose the bifurcation of the proper digital artery into the branches to the middle and ring fingers. Ligate and cut the branch to the ring finger a few millimeters from the bifurcation.

> Take great care in preventing damage to the vessel or excessive handling of the vessels as it may lead to spasm of the vessel.

10. Now the flap can be raised. Make the first incision on the mid-volar side. This incision must be down to the fibrous flexor sheath. There are a few transversely oriented subcutaneous volar veins at this area which must be cauterized. The volar portion of the flap can be raised now, up to the neutral line. The next incision should be made on the dorsal side down to the extensor paratenon and the dorsal portion of the flap raised. Now the distal margin of the flap incised and the neurovascular bundle ligated with 3.0 vicryl and cut. The flap is now attached by the Grayson's and Cleland's ligaments. To divide these, the flap must be lifted up, the neurovascular bundle confirmed to enter the flap and the ligaments must be divided close to the bone. This will free the flap some more.

11. Now make the incision marked on the ulnar neutral line and the marked proximal border of the flap. Care should be exercised, as the neurovascular bundle is deep to this area. Gently free the neurovascular bundle from the fibrous attachments and the multiple small branches coursing into the web. Now the flap is totally free, attached only at the pivot point "A" (Fig. 2.3.3).
12. Gently move the flap to the defect over the skin to check whether it reaches the defect comfortably (Fig. 2.3.4). If it does not, a little more dissection of the pedicle is in order.
13. Now develop a subcutaneous tunnel between the proximal edge of the defect and the pivot point of the flap. This tunnel should be created with the help of a tendon tunneller. The plane of the tunnel should be superficial to the palmar aponeurosis. This tunnel should be wide enough to hold the flap as it passes through, without traumatizing it.
14. Apply a stitch with 3.0 vicryl on the leading edge of the flap.
15. Apply wet gauze on the bed of the flap, xylocaine soaked gauze on the pedicle of the flap. Raise-up the hand and release the tourniquet. Maintain the hand in elevated position for about 3 minutes and ask for the tourniquet to be removed entirely.
16. Now set the hand on the table and examine the edges of the flap. There should be a slow and sustained subdermal bleed. This may not be evident immediately. It may take a few minutes for the spasm of the vessel to be relieved. In the meantime, continue to bathe the pedicle with 1 percent xylocaine solution and achieve hemostasis on the bed of the flap and the primary defect.

> If there is no bleeding from the flap edges, look for the following problems and correct them:
> - Any twist or kink in the vascular pedicle
> - Any ligature of a branch that is too close to the vessel.

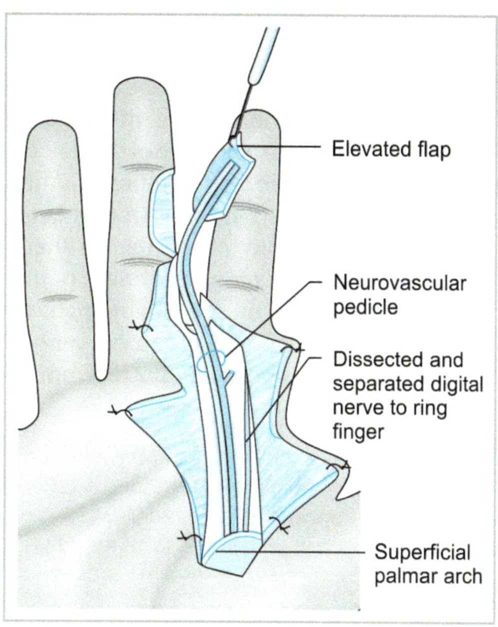

Fig. 2.3.3 Dissected flap

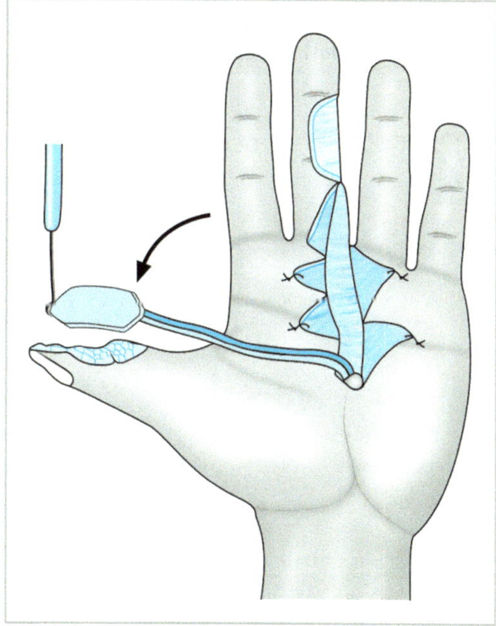

Fig. 2.3.4 Checking the reach

17. When good bleeding is seen from the edges of the flap, it is ready for transfer.
18. Pass a heavy curved hemostat from the proximal edge of the primary defect

through the tunnel. Grasp the 3.0 vicryl stitches that have been applied on the leading edge of the flap. Gently pull the hemostat with fine rocking movements and deliver the flap at the site of the defect. If it is difficult, redo step number 13. After delivering the flap in the wound site, confirm the viability of the flap. If there is reduced bleeding from the edges of the flap, the tunnel is most probably tight at the proximal edge which can be vented with a small incision of about 2 to 3 mm.

> This flap is usually a robust flap and there will be very brisk bleeding from the edges, especially after transfer. This is because the venous drainage takes time to regularize. So, get hemostasis on the edges of the flap before applying the insetting sutures!

19. *Flap inset:* After confirming the hemostasis and the viability of the flap, inset can be done with 4.0 ethilon using half buried horizontal mattress suturing (Fig. 2.3.5).

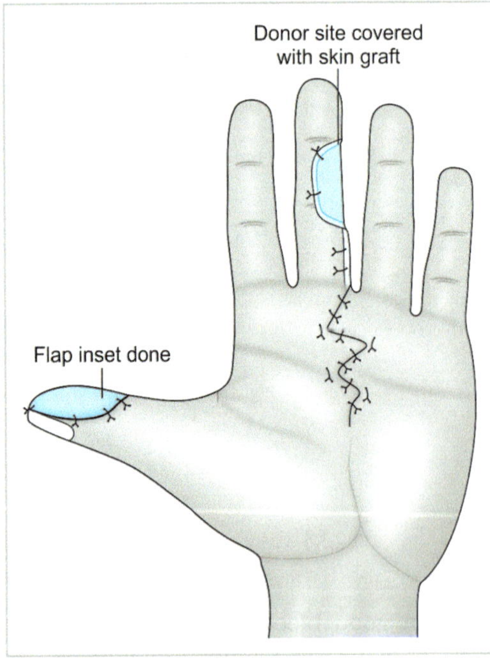

Fig. 2.3.5 After final flap inset and donor site closure with skin graft

20. *Management of the donor area:* After confirming hemostasis, the palmar flaps should be replaced and sutured with 4.0 ethilon. The residual raw area on the middle finger should be covered with a split thickness skin graft. At the points where the defect crosses the proximal interphalangeal (PIP) and DIP joint creases, back cuts should be given for 3 mm. to avoid skin graft contractures later on. Now raise the hand and prepare the arm with betadine solution. The skin graft should be harvested from the medial side of the arm. Sterile dressings should be applied over the skin graft donor site before moving back to the hand. The graft should be applied over the raw area and tie over sutures applied with 3.0 ethilon. Drainage tubes should be kept below the suture line on the palm of the hand. The preferred drainage tube would be Segmüller tube which consists of segments of the scalp vein set tubing.
21. Sterile dressings should be applied over the hand and the forearm. Care must be taken to avoid compression of the pedicle at any point of its course. A finger dressing must be applied on the middle finger and a short straightening splint should be applied on the volar side of the finger. A dorsal POP slab should be applied for the thumb keeping the wrist in neutral, and the metacarpophalangeal (MCP) joint of the thumb in flexion of 20° and interphalangeal (IP) joint in extension. A window must be made in the dressings to allow inspection and monitoring of the flap.

Postoperative Protocol

- Admission in the ward
- The affected hand should be kept elevated
- Patient can take normal diet immediately if the procedure was under regional block or after complete recovery if under general anesthesia

- Clinical monitoring of the flap once every 6 hours
- Analgesics and antibiotics for 5 days
- Sedation sos for 1 day
- Inspection of the dressing after 48 hours
- Discharge of the patient by 3rd day
- Suture removal on the 10th day and removal of donor site dressing on the arm
- Removal of the POP slab on the 14th day and advice the following:
- Refer to physiotherapy for active and passive mobilization of the thumb and fingers
- Daily wash with soap and water
- Massage of scar and grafted skin with coconut oil.
- Compression garment for scar softening after a further 2 weeks
- Sensory re-education exercises by physiotherapist.

First Dorsal Metacarpal Artery Flap

4

Introduction

First dorsal metacarpal artery flap is the flap of choice for defects on the dorsum of the thumb not extending beyond the level of the interphalangeal (IP) joint. The flap is based on the first dorsal metacarpal artery that usually arises from the radial artery at the level of the anatomical snuffbox.

Advantages of the Flap

- It is a single-staged procedure
- It is a sensate flap (because it is neurotized by the branches of the superficial branch of the radial nerve)
- Minimal morbidity in terms of donor site scarring.

Disadvantages of the Flap

- It is not very reliable (because of inconsistent anatomy)
- It requires expertise to raise this flap
- An alternate plan must always be ready.

Presurgical Counseling

- This procedure is planned to cover the raw area on the thumb with skin and tissues with sensation.
- This procedure will be done under axillary block anesthesia or GA in children.
- This procedure will take about 3 hours to perform.
- Skin will be removed along with soft tissues from the index finger and placed on the raw area of the thumb. This will entail making incisions on the back of the hand also. A skin graft will be taken from the medial side of the upper arm and applied over the secondary raw area on the index finger. There will be no deficit on the index finger, but there will be a scar on the finger. There will also be a scar on the medial side of the arm.
- Admission will be necessary for a minimum period of 3 days.
- A dressing will be applied and a plaster of Paris (POP) will be applied, which will be retained for 10 days, following which, physiotherapy will be started. The sensation that returns may not be equal to the sensation on the normal thumb.
- A splint will have to be applied on the index finger for a period of 3 to 4 weeks afterward.
- In some instances, the flap may not be possible because of anatomical variations. In such cases, other surgery like an abdominal flap may be done.
- The general complications of local anesthetic infiltration like hypersensitivity may occur in spite of test dose application. This complication will cause dryness of mouth and apprehension, which can be corrected immediately.

Surgical Steps

1. The preferred anesthesia is either axillary block or general anesthesia (in children).
2. Apply the tourniquet and keep ready.
3. Preparation and draping as described in Appendix I.
4. Raise the tourniquet and note the time.
5. Debride the defect and measure it. Make sure that the edges consist of intact and healthy skin. Take a lint pattern of the defect.
6. *Markings for the flap:*
   - Take the lint pattern and mark the flap on the dorsum of the proximal phalanx region of the index finger, just beyond the level of the knuckle. This is the "business end" of the flap. This flap is marked like a cross-finger flap. The distal limit of this flap is the dorsal proximal interphalangeal (PIP) joint line, the radial and ulnar limits are the respective neutral lines.
   - Mark a point exactly at the junction of the I metacarpal and the II metacarpal on the dorsum of the hand distal to the anatomical snuffbox. This is point A—the pivot point. This is the point where the first dorsal metacarpal artery arises from the radial artery.
   - Now mark the line of the II metacarpal bone on the skin.
   - Now mark a point on the radial side of the knuckle of the index finger. This is point B (Fig. 2.4.1) This point should lie on the proximal border of the marked flap and should also be radial to the distal end of the II metacarpal bone.
   - Join the points "A" and "B" with a gentle S-shaped line. This S-shaped line will have two curves: (1) a curve convex toward the radial side and (2) a curve convex toward the ulnar side. When marking the S-shaped line from the point "A" to "B", make sure that the curve convex to the radial side is proximal and the curve convex to the ulnar side is distal. This method reduces the distance between the pivot point and the defect.

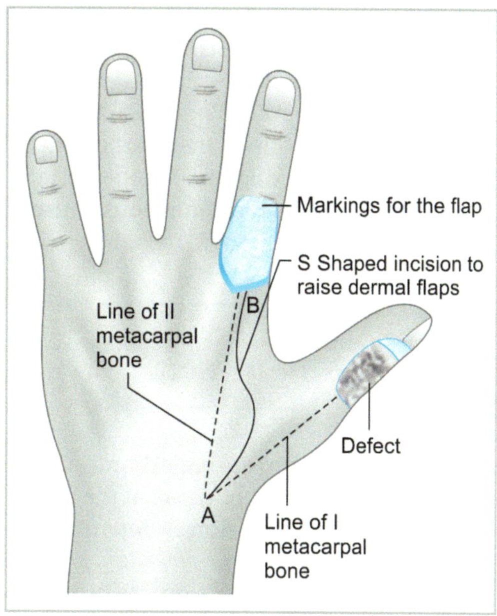

Fig. 2.4.1 Markings for the flap

7. Make the incision over the S-shaped line from "A" to "B". This incision should be only up to the dermis level, i.e. the incision should be made only to the depth where the underlying fat is just seen. Apply two skin hooks on the same side and elevate the dermal flaps on the radial side and then on the ulnar side. The flap should be raised on the radial side almost till the free margin of the thumb web and the I metacarpal bone. The flap on the ulnar side should be raised up to the entire length of the II metacarpal bone. Remember that the surgeon will not encounter the extensor tendons by this dissection. Anchor the dermal flaps with 3.0 nylon.
8. Now, what is exposed will be the subcutaneous tissue between the I and II metacarpal bones with the subcutaneous veins and the branches of the superficial radial nerve. Make an incision on the ulnar border of this tissue right over the II metacarpal bone, extending along the entire length of the bone. Raise this "flap" of subcutaneous tissue gently.

Underneath, the fascia covering the first dorsal interosseous muscle can be seen. Incise this fascia at its attachment to the II metacarpal bone. When this fascia is raised, the first dorsal metacarpal artery can be seen coursing on its undersurface and the first dorsal interosseous muscle belly can be seen.

> Try to include as many veins in the flap as possible. This will ensure good venous drainage of the flap.

9. Make an incision on the radial border of the subcutaneous "flap" of tissue at the radial border of the first dorsal interosseous muscle.
10. Now, make the incisions on the proximal phalangeal region of the index finger as marked. The distal, radial and ulnar edges should be incised down to the extensor paratenon (as is done for a cross-finger flap). When this is done, the flap will be attached only by the entire proximal border which has not been incised.
11. Make the incision of the proximal border as dermal flaps. Anchor these flaps too with 3.0 nylon.
12. Now, continue the incision made on the radial border of the first dorsal interosseous fascia in a distal direction. In this way, the radial side extensor expansion of the index finger will be encountered. Incise through this structure distally till the metacarpophalangeal (MCP) joint is crossed. This step ensures that the terminal end of the first dorsal metacarpal artery is not damaged during the dissection, as the tongue of extensor expansion protects it.
13. Now, the flap is lifted with skin hooks and raised off the bed. It will be noted that the distal portion of the flap contains only skin and subcutaneous tissue, proximally, it contains a segment of the extensor expansion and even further proximally, the superficial part of the first dorsal interosseous tendon and the fascia over this muscle with the first dorsal metacarpal artery on its undersurface and subcutaneous tissue containing the subcutaneous veins and the branches of the superficial radial nerve. Now, the flap has been raised totally (Fig. 2.4.2).
14. Now, develop a subcutaneous tunnel between the proximal edge of the defect and the pivot point of the flap. This tunnel should be created with the help of a tendon tunneller. This tunnel should be wide enough to hold the flap as it passes through, without traumatizing it.
15. Apply a stitch with 3.0 vicryl on the leading edge of the flap.
16. Apply wet gauze on the bed of the flap, xylocaine soaked gauze on the pedicle of the flap. Raise-up the hand and release the tourniquet. Maintain the hand in elevated position for about 3 minutes and ask for the tourniquet to be removed entirely.
17. Now, set the hand on the table and examine the edges of the flap. There should be a slow and sustained subdermal bleed. This may

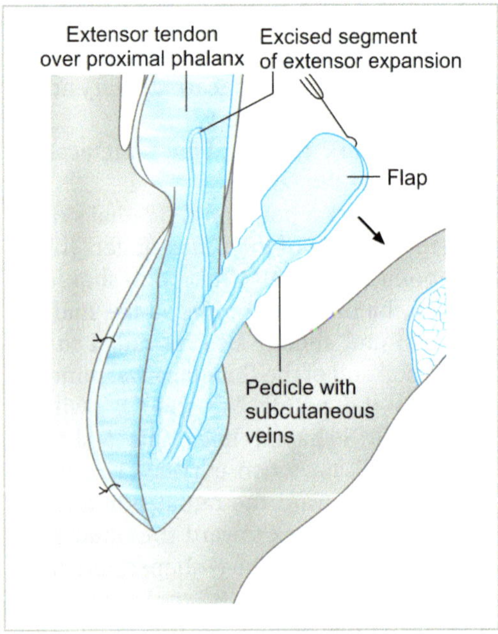

Fig. 2.4.2 Flap being raised

not be evident immediately. It may take a few minutes for the spasm of the vessel to be relieved. In the meantime, continue to bathe the pedicle with 1 percent xylocaine solution and achieve hemostasis on the bed of the flap and the primary defect.

18. When good bleeding is seen from the edges of the flap, it is ready for transfer.

> If there is no bleeding from the edges of the flap even after the waiting period, most probably, the flap may not survive. Now, the decision must be made whether to retain the flap and wait for a few days (which can be done if there is some bleed from the edges) or totally excise the flap, cover the donor site with a skin graft and plan for an abdominal flap cover for the primary raw area on the thumb.

19. Pass a heavy curved hemostat from the proximal edge of the primary defect through the tunnel. Grasp the 3.0 vicryl stitch that has been applied on the leading edge of the flap. Gently pull the hemostat with fine rocking movements and deliver the flap at the site of the defect. If it is difficult, redo step number 14. After delivering the flap in the wound site, confirm the viability of the flap. If there is reduced bleeding from the edges of the flap, the tunnel is most probably tight at the proximal edge which can be vented with a small incision of about 2 to 3 mm.
20. *Flap inset:* After confirming the hemostasis and the viability of the flap, inset can be done with 4.0 ethilon using half-buried horizontal mattress suturing.
21. *Management of the donor area:* After confirming hemostasis, the gap in the extensor expansion should first be repaired primarily with 4.0 polypropylene materials using horizontal mattress suture. The dermal flaps should be replaced and sutured with 4.0 ethilon. The residual raw area on the dorsum of the index finger should be covered with a split thickness skin graft (Fig. 2.4.3). Now raise the hand and prepare the arm with betadine solution. The skin graft should be harvested from the medial side of the arm. Sterile dressings should be applied over the skin graft donor site before moving back to the hand. The graft should be applied over the raw area and tie over sutures applied with 3.0 ethilon. Drainage tubes should be kept below the suture line on the dorsum of the hand. The preferred drainage tube would be Segmüller tube, which consists of segments of the scalp vein set tubing.

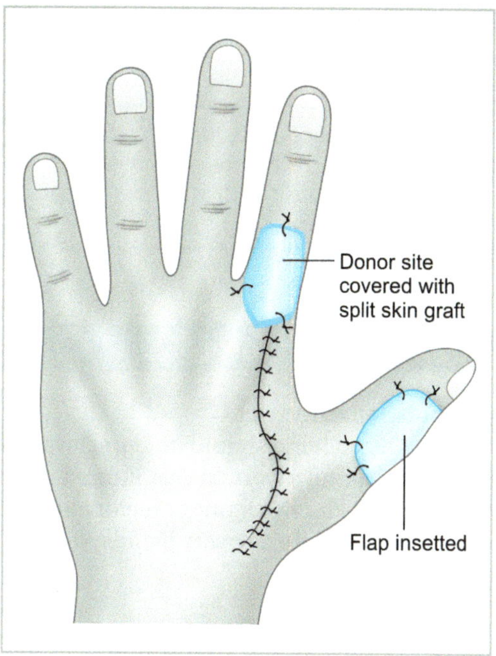

Fig. 2.4.3 After flap inset

22. Sterile dressings should be applied over the index finger, dorsum of hand and the thumb. Care must be taken to avoid compression of the pedicle at any point of its course. A volar POP slab should be applied for the thumb keeping it in palmar abduction and another slab for the hand keeping the MCP joints of the fingers in flexion of 90° and IP joints in extension. A window must be made in the dressings

to allow inspection and monitoring of the flap.

> If there is evidence of reduced blood flow in the flap postoperatively, the sutures should be removed immediately and all tension released from the suture line.

Postoperative Protocol

- Admission in the ward
- The affected hand should be kept elevated
- Patient can take normal diet immediately if the procedure was under regional block or after complete recovery if under general anesthesia
- Clinical monitoring of the flap once every 6 hours
- Analgesics and antibiotics for 5 days
- Sedation sos for 1 day
- Inspection of the dressing after 48 hours
- Discharge of the patient by 3rd day
- Suture removal on the 10th day and removal of donor site dressing on the arm
- Removal of the POP slab on the 14th day and advise the following:
    - Refer to physiotherapy for active and passive mobilization of the fingers and thumb
    - Daily wash with soap and water
    - Massage of scar and grafted skin with coconut oil
    - Compression garment for scar softening after a further 2 weeks.

5 Reverse Dorsal Metacarpal Artery Flap

Introduction

This flap is a useful flap in the armamentarium of the hand surgeon. It serves as an ideal skin cover for defects on the dorsum of the fingers on the proximal phalangeal region alone. The flap cannot cover defects that extend beyond the proximal interphalangeal (PIP) joint. Three dorsal metacarpal artery flaps are possible from the dorsum of the hand: the second, third and fourth dorsal metacarpal artery flaps. The second dorsal metacarpal artery flap can cover defects on the dorsum of the index or middle fingers. Similarly, the third dorsal metacarpal artery flap can cover defects on the dorsum of the middle or ring fingers, and the fourth dorsal metacarpal artery flap can be used for defects on the ring or little fingers.

This flap can be planned only if two criteria are met:

1. The width of the flap should be such that primary closure of the defect must be possible on the dorsum of the hand. This can be assessed by pinching up a fold of skin on the dorsum of the hand.
2. The length of the flap should not extend beyond the dorsal wrist crease.

Advantages of the Flap

- It is a single stage procedure

Disadvantages of the Flap

- It is not a very reliable flap as there are many anatomic variations
- It is a reverse flow flap and hence, like all reverse flow flaps, is prone for venous congestion.
- There is considerable donor site morbidity.

Presurgical Counseling

- This procedure is planned to cover the raw area on the finger with skin and tissues.
- This procedure will be done under axillary block anesthesia.
- This procedure will take about 3 hours to perform.
- Skin will be removed along with soft tissues from the back of the hand and placed on the raw area on the finger. There will be a scar on the back of the hand.
- Admission will be necessary for a minimum period of 3 days.
- A dressing will be applied and a plaster of Paris (POP) will be applied, which will be retained for 10 days, following which, physiotherapy will be started
- In some instances, the flap may not be possible because of anatomical variations. In such cases, other surgery like a cross-finger flap may be done
- The general complications of local anesthetic infiltration like hypersensitivity

may occur in spite of test dose application. This complication will cause dryness of mouth and apprehension, which can be corrected immediately.

Surgical Steps

1. The preferred anesthesia is either axillary block or general anesthesia (in children)
2. Apply the tourniquet and keep ready
3. Preparation and draping as described in Appendix I
4. Raise the tourniquet and note the time
5. Debride the defect and measure it. Make sure that the edges consist of intact and healthy skin. Take a lint pattern of the defect
6. *Markings for the flap (Fig. 2.5.1):*
   - Mark the two knuckle prominences corresponding to the flap that has been chosen. If the second dorsal metacarpal artery flap has been chosen, the knuckles of the index and middle fingers are the landmarks. If the third dorsal metacarpal artery flap has been decided on, the middle and ring finger knuckle prominences form the landmarks. Similarly, the knuckle prominences of the ring and little fingers are the landmarks if the fourth dorsal metacarpal artery flap has been chosen.
   - Mark a point "A" about 1 cm proximal to the knuckle prominences. This point forms the pivot point of the dorsal metacarpal artery flap.
   - Measure the distance between the points "A" and the proximal border of the defect. This distance is the length of the pedicle
   - Transpose this distance proximal to the point "A" on the dorsum of the hand and mark this point as "B". Place the lint pattern with its proximal border at point "B" and make the marking of the flap. When this is done, the distal end of the flap marking "C" must not extend beyond the wrist joint line
   - Mark two parallel lines on either side of the line "AB", about 1 cm away. This will be the width of the subcutaneous pedicle. The distal ends of these lines will cut the proximal border of the flap at points "D" and "E".
7. Now, make the incision "DCE". This incision must go through the skin and subcutaneous tissue to the level of the extensor paratenon, which is the thin filmy layer over the extensor tendon. Do not injure this paratenon. Raise the flap superficial to this structure. The subcutaneous veins that cross the incision should be divided and ligated.
8. Now, make the incisions "EBD" and "BA". These incisions should be superficial just through the epidermis and dermis, to expose the fat underneath. Place skin hooks and raise the dermal flaps on the radial side and on the ulnar side till the marked area. Apply anchoring sutures with 3.0 ethilon. You will be able to see fibrofatty tissue in the bed, containing a few subcutaneous veins. These veins

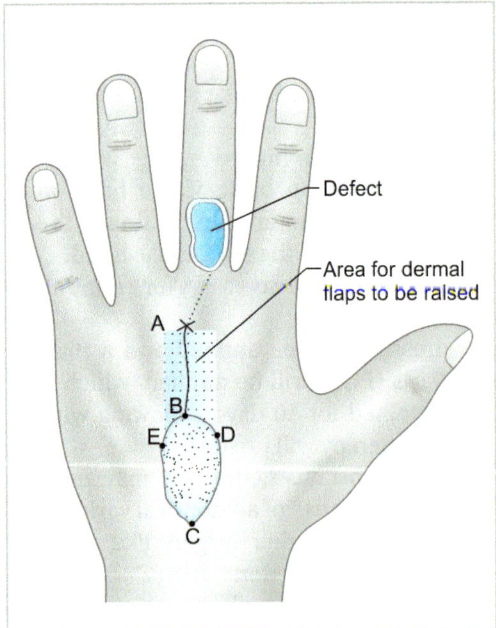

Fig. 2.5.1 Flap markings

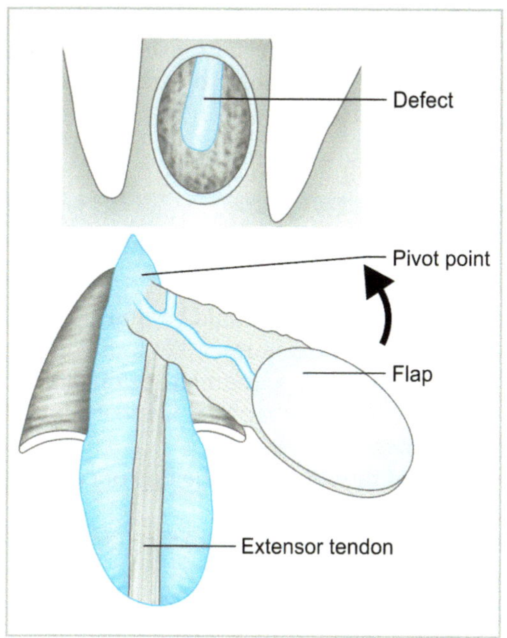

Fig. 2.5.2 Flap after elevation

are important to ensure good venous drainage for the flap. Incise the fascia at the marked area. Now, lift the distal edge of the flap with skin hooks and elevate the flap off the bed. This dissection should stop at point "A". The flap has now been elevated (Fig. 2.5.2).

9. Now, develop a subcutaneous tunnel between the proximal edge of the defect and the pivot point of the flap. This tunnel should be created with the help of a tendon tunneller. This tunnel should be wide enough to hold the flap as it passes through, without traumatizing it.
10. Apply a stitch with 3.0 nylon on the leading edge of the flap.
11. Apply wet gauze on the bed of the flap, xylocaine soaked gauze on the pedicle of the flap. Raise-up the hand and release the tourniquet. Maintain the hand in elevated position for about 3 minutes and ask for the tourniquet to be removed entirely.
12. Now, set the hand on the table and examine the edges of the flap. There should be a slow and sustained subdermal bleed. This may not be evident immediately. It may take a few minutes for the spasm of the vessel to be relieved. In the meantime, continue to bathe the pedicle with 1 percent xylocaine solution and achieve hemostasis on the bed of the flap and the primary defect.
13. When good bleeding is seen from the edges of the flap, it is ready for transfer.
14. Pass a heavy curved hemostat from the proximal edge of the primary defect through the tunnel. Grasp the 3.0 vicryl stitch that has been applied on the leading edge of the flap. Gently pull the hemostat with fine rocking movements and deliver the flap at the site of the defect. If it is difficult, redo step 14. After delivering the flap in the wound site, confirm the viability of the flap.

The most common reasons why this flap sometimes undergoes vascular compromise are the following reasons:

- Tightness of the tunnel as mentioned
- Tight inset of the flap edges to the edges of the defect
- If there is tightness of the tunnel, the tunnel is most probably tight at the proximal edge which can be vented with a small incision of about 2–3 mm
- If there is tightness of the suture line of the inset, remove the sutures on one side—either the radial or ulnar side and cover this exposed area with a skin graft.

15. *Flap inset:* After confirming the hemostasis and the viability of the flap, inset can be done with 4.0 ethilon using half buried horizontal mattress suturing.
16. *Management of the donor area:* After confirming hemostasis, the defect should first be closed primarily with 4.0 polypropylene materials using vertical mattress suture. The dermal flaps should be replaced and sutured with 4.0 ethilon (Fig. 2.5.3). Drainage tubes should be kept below the suture line on the dorsum of the hand. The preferred drainage tube would be Segmüller tube which consists of segments of the scalp vein set tubing.

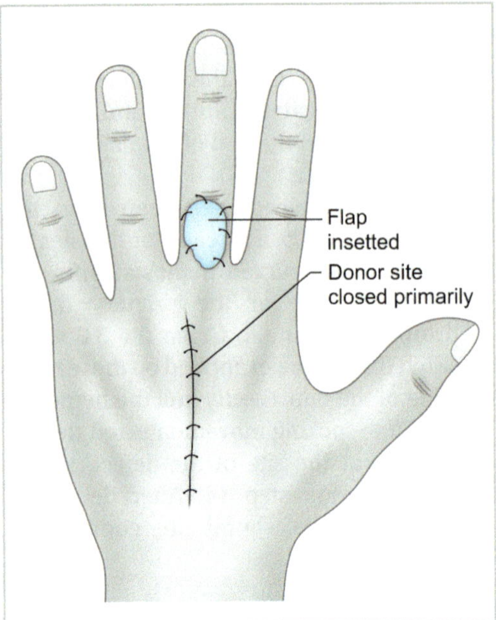

Fig. 2.5.3 After flap inset and management of the donor site

17. Sterile dressings should be applied over the index finger, dorsum of hand. Care must be taken to avoid compression of the pedicle at any point of its course. A volar POP slab should be applied for the hand keeping the metacarpophalangeal (MCP) joints of the fingers in flexion of 90° and interphalangeal (IP) joints in extension. A window must be made in the dressings to allow inspection and monitoring of the flap, extending from the distal most point of the flap to the pivot point of the flap.

Postoperative Protocol

- Admission in the ward
- The affected hand should be kept elevated
- Patient can take normal diet immediately if the procedure was under regional block or after complete recovery if under general anesthesia
- Clinical monitoring of the flap once every 6 hours
- Analgesics and antibiotics for 5 days
- Sedation sos for 1 day
- Inspection of the dressing after 48 hours
- Discharge of the patient by 3rd day
- Suture removal on the 10th day and removal of donor site dressing on the arm
- Removal of the POP slab on the 14th day and advise the following:
    - Refer to physiotherapy for active and passive mobilization of the fingers and thumb
    - Daily wash with soap and water
    - Massage of scar and grafted skin with coconut oil
    - Compression garment for scar softening after a further 2 weeks.

Posterior Interosseous Artery Flap

6

Introduction

The posterior interosseous flap is a reverse flow flap based on the posterior interosseous artery.

Indications

- Defects on the dorsum of hand with no tendon injury
- Defects on the dorsum of hand and a single finger not extending beyond the proximal interphalangeal (PIP) joint
- Defects on the ulnar border of the hand
- Defect on the thumb web or dorsum of the thumb
- Defects on the flexor aspect of the wrist.

Advantages

- It is a single-staged procedure
- Reliable flap
- Same field of regional block anesthesia.

Disadvantages

- Brings hair bearing skin to the hand
- Donor site morbidity is high
- Requires expertise.

Presurgical Counseling

- This procedure is planned to cover the raw area with skin and tissues
- This procedure will be done under axillary block anesthesia (except for children, in whom general anesthesia may be required) with a short general anesthesia while harvesting a skin graft from the thigh
- This procedure will take about 3 hours to perform
- Skin will be removed along with soft tissues from the back of the forearm and placed on the raw area. A skin graft will be taken from the medial side of the thigh and applied over the secondary raw area on the forearm. There will be no deficit on the forearm, but there will be a scar on the forearm. There will consequently be a scar on the thigh also
- Admission will be necessary for a minimum period of 3 days
- A dressing will be applied and a plaster of Paris (POP) will be applied, which will be retained for 10 days, following which, physiotherapy will be started
- In some instances, the flap may not be possible because of anatomical variations. In such cases, other surgery like an abdominal/groin flap may have to be done.
- In rare instances, after the flap has been done, there may be a problem to the vascularity and the flap may necrose. In such cases, other surgery like an abdominal

or groin flap may be required to be done later
- The general complications of local anesthetic infiltration like hypersensitivity may occur in spite of test dose application. This complication will cause dryness of mouth and apprehension, which can be corrected immediately.

Surgical Steps

1. The preferred anesthesia is either axillary block or general anesthesia (in children).
2. Apply the tourniquet and keep ready.
3. Preparation and draping as described in Appendix I.
4. The elbow area must also be prepared and kept exposed.
5. Raise the tourniquet and note the time.
6. Debride the defect and measure it. Make sure that the edges consist of intact and healthy skin. Take a lint pattern of the defect.
7. *Markings for the flap (Fig. 2.6.1):* Mark the following points on the extensor aspect of the forearm (the markings must be made before the tourniquet is raised):
    - Point "A"—radial styloid
    - Point "B"—head of ulna
    - Join points "A" and "B"
    - Mark a point "C" at the junction of ulnar one-third and radial two-thirds of line AB. This represents the point where the posterior interosseous artery anastomoses with the terminal end of the anterior interosseous artery.
    - Mark a point "D" exactly over the lateral epicondyle.
    - Join the points "C" and "D". This represents the axis of the flap, i.e. the course of the posterior interosseous artery, even though the origin of the artery is about 8 cm distal to point "D".
    - Mark a point "E" about 2 cm proximal to point "C", on the line CD. This will represent the distal most point of our dissection
    - Mark the mid-point "F" of the line CD. Mark another point "X, 1 cm distal to the point "F". This point "X" represents the point at which the central cutaneous perforator of the posterior interosseous artery appears. This point must be included in the flap (Fig. 2.6.2).
    - Now, measure the distance between the point "E" and the proximal edge of the defect. This will represent the length of the pedicle. Transpose this distance on the line ED and mark the point as "G". Place the lint pattern of the defect centered on the axis DE, with its proximal edge at the point "G". Make sure that the flap covers the point "X". Also make sure that the proximal border is at least 6 cm distal to point "D".
    - Draw a transverse line 2 cm proximal to the point "X" to meet the radial and ulnar sides of the marked flap at "H" and "I" respectively. Draw two lines 2 cm parallel to the line CG, one on the radial side and one on the ulnar side. These lines represent the limit of dissection on the radial and ulnar sides. These lines will cut the marking of the flap at the points "J" and "K" on the radial and ulnar sides respectively.

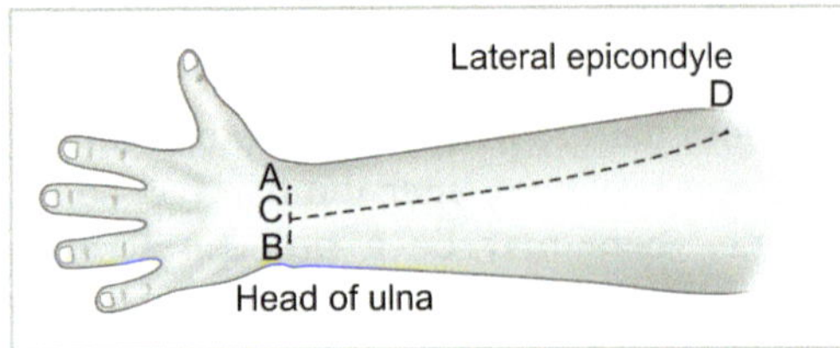

Fig. 2.6.1 Preliminary markings

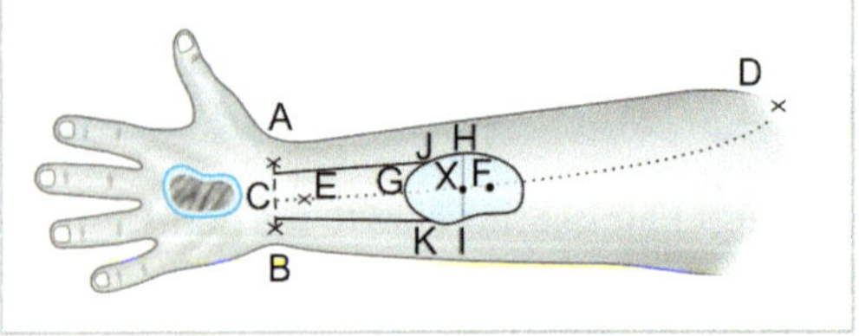

Fig. 2.6.2 Final markings of the flap

8. Make the incision from "J" to "K" on the proximal border. This incision should be down to the deep fascia only. Do not incise the deep fascia. Secure hemostasis as there are many veins crossing the incision. After making the incision, raise this flap as a skin flap, superficial to the thick white layer of the deep fascia. The deeper muscles can be visualized at this stage under the fascia. Starting from the ulna, the first compartment (not to be confused with extensor compartments at the dorsum of the wrist) seen is the extensor carpi ulnaris (ECU) muscle. The next big compartment is the extensor digitorum communis (EDC). Between these two compartments, a new compartment starts forming at about 6 to 8 cm from the lateral epicondyle. This is the extensor digiti minimi (EDM) muscle. Stop at the marked line HI. Now, raise the remaining portion of the flap first from the ulnar side (IK). As it is raised superficial to the deep fascia, stop when you cross the ulna bone. Once the ulna is crossed, deepen the incision by incising the deep fascia. The ECU muscle will be seen. With gentle radialward retraction of the flap, identify the radial border of the muscle and stop. Similarly, raise the radial portion (HJ) till the muscle compartment of the EDM muscle is identified underneath the deep fascia. Deepen the incision through the deep fascia at the radial edge of the muscle. With gentle ulnarward traction on the flap identifies the ulnar border of the muscle and retracts the muscle radialward. Now the posterior interosseous vascular pedicle along with the terminal branches of the posterior interosseous nerve will be seen at the depth of the intermuscular septum between the EDM and ECU muscles. The perforator from the posterior interosseous artery to the skin can also be seen reaching the skin at the level of our marking "X".
9. Identify the posterior interosseous nerve and separate it from the vascular pedicle. There is usually a thin fascia covering the neurovascular bundle. This will have to be opened to facilitate dissection. Dissect the posterior interosseous artery and ligate the branches to the muscles. Now, ligate and divide the posterior interosseous artery and veins proximal to the central perforator, making sure that the nerve has been safeguarded.

> This dissection is easily carried out on the radial side (Fig. 2.6.3), i.e. from the EDM muscle side by retracting the muscle, rather than the ECU side. Avoid injuring the posterior interosseous nerve at this juncture.

10. Now make the incision on the line GD. This must be a superficial incision, just through the epidermis and dermis, to expose the fat underneath. Place skin hooks and raise the dermal flaps on the radial side and on the ulnar side till the marked area. Apply anchoring sutures with 3.0 ethilon. You will be able to see fibrofatty tissue in the bed, containing a few subcutaneous veins. These veins are important to ensure good venous drainage for the flap. Make the incisions on this tissue at the radial and ulnar ends (along the marked limits of dissection). These incisions can go deep to the fascia.

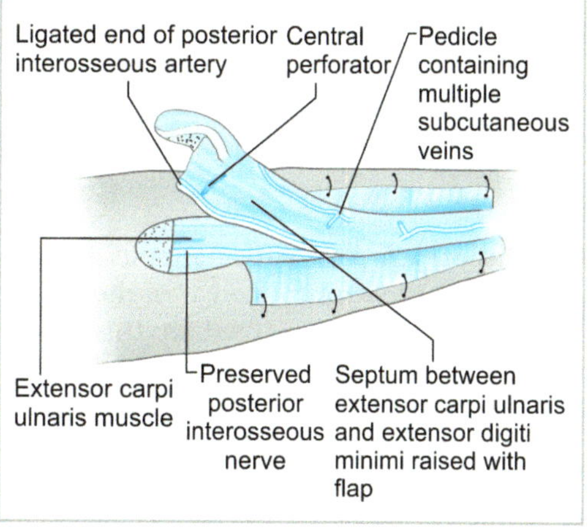

Fig. 2.6.3 View of the raised flap (from the radial side)

Retract the EDM muscle radially and the ECU muscle ulnarly and the entire course of the posterior interosseous vessels can be seen.

Try to get as many veins in the subcutaneous tissues. It does not matter if the veins have been accidentally damaged or cauterized. It is only the venous channels that serve to drain the flap by the help of intervenous channels.

11. Lift-up the flap and divide the intermuscular septum deep to the level of the posterior interosseous vessels. As you keep advancing, make sure to cauterize or ligate the muscular branches.

    Keep ensuring that no damage occurs to the vascular pedicle. When we encounter some small branches to the ulna bone, it means we have come close to the pivot point. In this way, the flap can be raised up to the level of the point "D". At this level, the vessels will lie between the ECU and EDM tendons.

    Transpose the flap to the defect to approximately see whether the flap covers the defect (Fig. 2.6.4). If it does not do so, elevate the pedicle a little more.

This is fondly called the "heart attack point" (for the surgeon). This is because the vessel becomes so small, that it is no longer visualized in the dissected pedicle tissue. Hence, the chances of injury to the vessel are high. The way to avoid injury to the vessels at this level is to raise the pedicle tissue very close to the ulna bone which lies underneath.

12. Now, develop a subcutaneous tunnel between the proximal edge of the defect and the pivot point of the flap. This tunnel should be created with the help of a tendon tunneller. This tunnel should be wide enough to hold the flap as it passes through, without traumatizing it.
13. Apply a stitch with 3.0 vicryl on the leading edge of the flap.

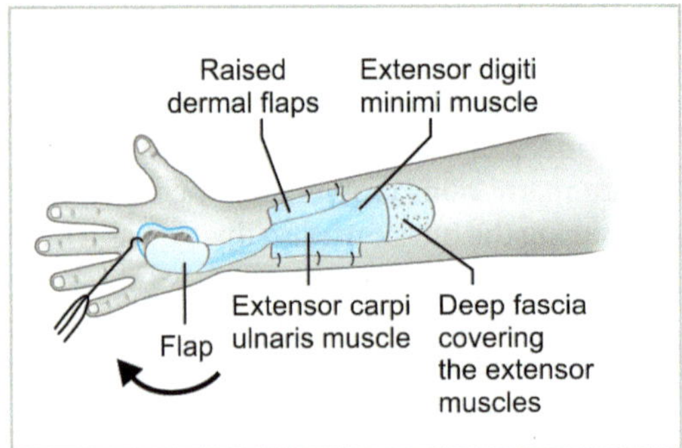

Fig. 2.6.4 Checking the reach of the flap

14. Apply wet gauze on the bed of the flap, xylocaine soaked gauze on the pedicle of the flap. Raise-up the hand and release the tourniquet. Maintain the hand in elevated position for about 3 minutes and ask for the tourniquet to be removed entirely.
15. Now, set the hand on the table and examine the edges of the flap. There should be a slow and sustained subdermal bleed. This may not be evident immediately. It may take a few minutes for the spasm of the vessel to be relieved. In the meantime, continue to bathe the pedicle with 1 percent xylocaine solution and achieve hemostasis on the bed of the flap and the primary defect.

This flap is usually a robust flap and there will be good bleeding from the edges. Before transferring the flap, turn the flap raw side up and get hemostasis on the pedicle carefully!

16. When good bleeding is seen from the edges of the flap, it is ready for transfer.
17. Pass a heavy curved hemostat from the proximal edge of the primary defect through the tunnel. Grasp the 3.0 vicryl stitch that has been applied on the leading edge of the flap. Gently pull the hemostat with fine rocking movements and deliver the flap at the site of the defect. If it is difficult, redo step 14. After delivering the

flap in the wound site, confirm the viability of the flap. If there is reduced bleeding from the edges of the flap, the tunnel is most probably tight at the proximal edge which can be vented with a small incision of about 2 to 3 mm.

18. *Flap inset:* After confirming the hemostasis and the viability of the flap, inset can be done with 4.0 ethilon using half buried horizontal mattress suturing.
19. *Management of the donor area:* After confirming hemostasis, the dermal flaps should be replaced and sutured with 4.0 ethilon. The residual raw area on the extensor aspect of the forearm should be narrowed with 3.0 vicryl. Now prepare the thigh with betadine solution. The skin graft should be harvested from the medial side of the thigh. Sterile dressings should be applied over the skin graft donor site before moving back to the hand. The graft should be applied over the raw area and tie over sutures applied with 3.0 ethilon. Drainage tubes should be kept below the suture line on the forearm. The preferred drainage tube would be Segmüller tube which consists of segments of the scalp vein set tubing.
20. Sterile dressings should be applied over the hand and the forearm. Care must be taken to avoid compression of the pedicle at any point of its course. A volar POP slab should be applied for the hand keeping the wrist in 30° extension, and the metacarpophalangeal (MCP) joints of the fingers in flexion of 90° and interphalangeal (IP) joints in extension. A window must be made in the dressings to allow inspection and monitoring of the flap.

Inspect the flap after 6 hours. This is a critical period in the phase of the flap when the venous drainage has become established. However, there may be a hematoma due to bleeding in the interim period, and this may compress the vascular pedicle. If so, removal of one or two sutures and gentle compression to evacuate the hematoma will restore equilibrium in the flap.

Postoperative Protocol

- Admission in the ward
- The affected hand should be kept elevated
- Patient can take normal diet immediately if the procedure was under regional block or after complete recovery if under general anesthesia
- Clinical monitoring of the flap once every 6 hours
- Analgesics and antibiotics for 5 days
- Sedation sos for 1 day
- Inspection of the dressing after 48 hours
- Discharge of the patient by 3rd day
- Suture removal on the 10th day and removal of donor site dressing on the arm
- Removal of the POP slab on the 14th day and advice the following:
    - Refer to physiotherapy for active and passive mobilization of the fingers and thumb
    - Daily wash with soap and water
    - Massage of scar and grafted skin with coconut oil
    - Compression garment for scar softening after a further 2 weeks.

Radial Artery Forearm Flap

7

Introduction

Radial artery forearm flap is one of the versatile flaps being used in hand surgery ever since it was described by the Chinese. It can be used as a pedicled flap or as a free flap. In this chapter, its use as a pedicled flap is described. When used as a pedicled flap, it is a reverse flow flap.

Advantages

- It is a single staged procedure
- It brings a large amount of skin on to the hand.

Disadvantages

- It involves the sacrifice of a major artery of the upper limb
- It leaves a very bad scar on the forearm.

Presurgical Counseling

- This procedure is planned to cover the raw area with skin and tissues.
- This procedure will be done under axillary block anesthesia, with a short general anesthesia while harvesting a skin graft from the thigh.
- This procedure will take about 3 hours to perform.
- Skin will be removed along with soft tissues from the forearm and placed on the raw area. A skin graft will be taken from the medial side of the thigh and applied over the secondary raw area on the forearm. There will be no deficit on the forearm, but there will be a scar on the forearm. There will consequently be a scar on the thigh also.
- Admission will be necessary for a minimum period of 3 days.
- A dressing will be applied and a plaster of Paris (POP) will be applied, which will be retained for 10 days, following which, physiotherapy will be started.
- In some instances, the flap may not be possible because of anatomical variations. In such cases, other surgery like an abdominal or groin flap may be done.
- In rare instances, after the flap has been done, there may be a problem to the vascularity and the flap may necrose. In such cases, other surgery like an abdominal or groin flap may be done later.
- The general complications of local anesthetic infiltration like hypersensitivity may occur in spite of test dose application. This complication will cause dryness of mouth and apprehension, which can be corrected immediately.

Surgical Steps

1. The preferred anesthesia is either axillary block or general anesthesia (in children).
2. Apply the tourniquet and keep ready.

3. Preparation and draping as described in Appendix I.
4. The elbow area must also be prepared and kept exposed.
5. Raise the tourniquet and note the time.
6. Debride the defect and measure it. Make sure that the edges consist of intact and healthy skin. Take a lint pattern of the defect.
7. *Markings for the flap (Fig. 2.7.1):*
    - Draw a point "A" on the distal most palpable pulsation of the radial artery proximal to the wrist.
    - Mark a point "B" on the palpable biceps tendon in front of the elbow.
    - Join the points "A" and "B". This forms the axis of the flap.
    - Mark a point "C" about 2 cm proximal to point "A" on the line AB. This will represent the distal most point of our dissection.
    - Now measure the distance between the point "C" and the proximal edge of the defect. This will represent the length of the pedicle. Transpose this distance on the line AB and mark the point as "D". Place the lint pattern of the defect centered on the axis AB, with its proximal edge at the point "D". Mark the flap. Mark the distal most point on the flap as "G".
    - Draw two lines 2 cm parallel to the line CD, one on the radial side and one on the ulnar side. These lines represent the limit of dissection of the subcutaneous cuff on the radial and ulnar sides. These lines will cut the marking of the flap at the points "E" and "F" respectively on the radial and ulnar sides.

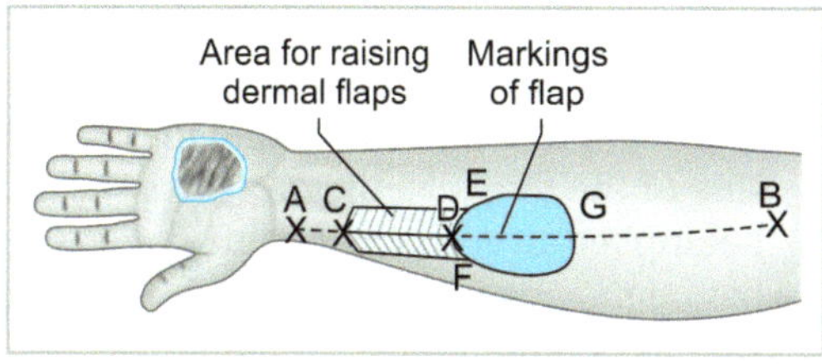

Fig. 2.7.1 Markings for the flap

8. Make the incision on the ulnar border of the flap from "G" to "F". This incision should be down to the level of the deep fascia of the forearm. Raise the flap superficial to the deep fascia, till the ulnar border of the flexor carpi radialis muscle is seen below the fascia. Now, deepen the incision and divide the deep fascia. Now continue raising the flap over the muscle, while applying gentle radialward and upward traction on the flap. Along the radial border of the muscle, the radial vascular bundle can be seen lying in a septum. Do not dissect on this septum now. Keep dissecting close to the muscle only. Apply a retractor on the radial border of the flexor carpi radialis muscle and retract it toward the ulnar side. This will expose the small branches of the radial artery to the flexor muscles. Carefully divide them away from the radial artery and secure hemostasis.
9. Now make the incision on the radial side from "G" to "E". Raise this flap superficial to the deep fascia. In this way we can avoid injury to the superficial branch of the radial nerve. Deepen the incision when the ulnar border of the brachioradialis muscle is seen beneath the fascia. Now raise the flap off the muscle by applying gentle ulnarward and upward traction on the flap. The radial vascular bundle can now be seen on the radial border of the muscle and its tendon. Apply a retractor on the ulnar border of the brachioradialis muscle and retract it toward the radial side. This will expose the small branches of the radial artery to the muscles. Carefully divide them away from the radial artery and secure hemostasis.
10. Now make the incision on the lines flexor digitorum communis (FDC) and extensor digitorum communis (EDC). These must be superficial incisions, just through the epidermis and dermis, to expose the fat underneath. Place skin hooks and raise the dermal flaps on the radial side and on the ulnar side till the marked area. Apply

anchoring sutures with 3.0 ethilon. You will be able to see fibrofatty tissue in the bed, containing a few subcutaneous veins including the cephalic vein. These veins are important to ensure good venous drainage for the flap. Make the incisions on this fatty subcutaneous tissue at the radial and ulnar ends (along the marked limits of dissection). These incisions can go deep to the fascia. Retract the brachioradialis tendon radially and the flexor carpi radialis tendon ulnarly and the entire course of the radial vessels can be seen.

11. Now go to the point "G" of the flap. Apply 2 ligatures with 3.0 vicryl at the proximal most point of the exposed radial vessels. Divide the vessels between the ligatures. Lift-up the flap gently and divide the septum deep to the level of the radial vessels, taking care to cauterize the deeper branches from the vessels.
12. Continue this dissection up to the point "C". Now the flap has been mobilized.
13. Now develop a subcutaneous tunnel between the proximal edge of the defect and the pivot point "C" of the flap. This tunnel should be created with the help of a tendon tunneller. This tunnel should be wide enough to hold the flap as it passes through, without traumatizing it.

It may not be possible to tunnel the palmar skin because this skin is thicker and more anchored to the subcutaneous tissues than the dorsal skin. In such situations, it may be ideal to make an incision on the palmar skin along the proposed track of the flap. This incision will be made through the skin and subcutaneous tissues, and both edges of the skin retracted to accommodate the pedicle. This will cause an unsightly scar on the palm. This may have to be excised later and the skin closed primarily to minimize the scar.

14. Apply a stitch with 3.0 nylon on the leading edge of the flap.
15. Apply wet gauze on the bed of the flap, xylocaine soaked gauze on the pedicle of the flap. Raise-up the hand and release the tourniquet. Maintain the hand in elevated position for about 3 minutes and ask for the tourniquet to be removed entirely.
16. Now set the hand on the table and examine the edges of the flap. There should be a slow and sustained subdermal bleed. This may not be evident immediately. It may take a few minutes for the spasm of the vessel to be relieved. In the meantime, continue to bathe the pedicle with 1 percent xylocaine solution and achieve hemostasis on the bed of the flap and the primary defect.
17. When good bleeding is seen from the edges of the flap, it is ready for transfer.
18. Pass a heavy curved hemostat from the proximal edge of the primary defect through the tunnel. Grasp the 3.0 vicryl stitch that has been applied on the leading edge of the flap. Gently pull the hemostat with fine rocking movements and deliver the flap at the site of the defect. After delivering the flap in the wound site, confirm the viability of the flap. If there is reduced bleeding from the edges of the flap, the tunnel is most probably tight at the proximal edge which can be vented with a small incision of about 2 to 3 mm.
19. *Flap inset:* After confirming the hemostasis and the viability of the flap, inset can be done with 4.0 ethilon using half buried horizontal mattress suturing.
20. *Management of the donor area (Fig. 2.7.2):* After confirming hemostasis, the dermal flaps should be replaced and sutured with 4.0 ethilon. The residual raw area on the extensor aspect of the forearm should be narrowed with 3.0 vicryl. Now prepare the thigh with betadine solution. The skin graft should be harvested from the medial side of the thigh. Sterile dressings should be applied over the skin graft donor site before moving back to the hand. The graft should be applied over the raw area and tie over sutures applied with 3.0 ethilon.

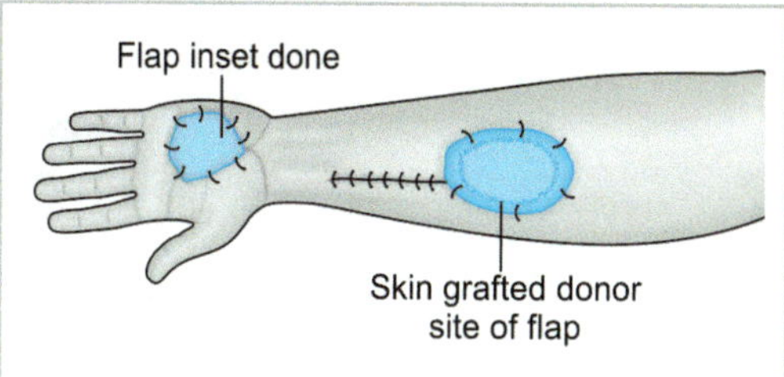

Fig. 2.7.2 Management of donor site

Drainage tubes should be kept below the suture line on the forearm. The preferred drainage tube would be Segmüller tube which consists of segments of the scalp vein set tubing.

21. Sterile dressings should be applied over the hand and the forearm. Care must be taken to avoid compression of the pedicle at any point of its course. A volar POP slab should be applied for the hand keeping the wrist in 30° extension, and the metacarpophalangeal (MCP) joints of the fingers in flexion of 90° and interphalangeal (IP) joints in extension. A window must be made in the dressings to allow inspection and monitoring of the flap.

Postoperative Protocol

- Admission in the ward
- The affected hand should be kept elevated.
- Patient can take normal diet immediately if the procedure was under regional block or after complete recovery if under general anesthesia.
- Clinical monitoring of the flap once every 6 hours.
- Analgesics and antibiotics for 5 days
- Sedation sos for 1 day
- Inspection of the dressing after 48 hours
- Discharge of the patient by 3rd day
- Suture removal on the 10th day and removal of donor site dressing on the arm
- *Removal of the POP slab on the 14th day and advice the following:*
    - Refer to physiotherapy for active and passive mobilization of the fingers and thumb.
    - Daily wash with soap and water.
    - Massage of scar and grafted skin with coconut oil.
    - Compression garment for scar softening after a further 2 weeks.

Buried Abdominal Flap

8

Introduction

Buried abdominal flap is the flap of choice for degloving injuries of the entire hand. Routinely used abdominal flaps and groin flaps are not enough to resurface such large areas and hence a different technique will have to be employed. The technique of using the buried abdominal flap refers to the method where the entire hand is buried in a pocket in the abdominal wall and then removed for further reconstruction. When the hand is buried in this manner in the abdominal wall, skin will still not be available to cover the entire hand. After the removal of the hand from the buried status in the abdominal wall, the further reconstruction may be of two types:

1. *Partial Crane technique:* The abdominal skin can be retained on the dorsal aspect of the hand and the residual raw area on the palmar aspect can be covered with skin graft, applied over the soft tissues (Crane principle).
2. *Full Crane technique:* An alternative method is to retain the abdominal skin in the abdomen and remove the hand with only the soft tissues covering it. This raw area is subsequently skin grafted.

Both these techniques have been described here:

Presurgical Counseling

- This procedure is planned to cover the entire raw area on the hand.
- This procedure will be done under axillary block anesthesia for the hand and either spinal anesthesia or general anesthesia.
- This procedure will take about 3 hours to perform.
- Incisions will be made on the abdominal wall and the entire hand bereft of skin will be buried in a pocket in the abdominal wall. This will be retained for a period of 2 weeks.
- After a period of 2 weeks, a delay procedure may have to be done under local anesthesia or spinal anesthesia.
- Admission will be necessary for a minimum period of 1 month.
- After the hand is removed from its buried position in the abdomen, a skin grafting will be required.
- There will be a scar in the abdominal wall.
- Splints and physiotherapy in the form of exercises will be required afterward
- The general complications of local anesthetic infiltration like hypersensitivity may occur in spite of test dose application. This complication will cause dryness of mouth and apprehension, which can be corrected immediately. Complications of general anesthesia or spinal anesthesia may occur.

Surgical Steps

1. The preferred anesthesia is axillary block and regional block or general anesthesia.
2. Apply the tourniquet and keep ready.

3. Preparation and draping as described in Appendix I.
4. Raise the tourniquet and note the time.
5. Debride the defect and measure it. Make sure that the edges consist of intact and healthy skin.
6. If all the fingers have been degloved, it is useful to disarticulate the fingers at the distal interphalangeal (DIP) joints, as the reconstruction and rehabilitation will be quicker and better.
7. *Markings for the flap:*
   - There are usually two types of total degloving injuries of the hand: (1) involves the thumb and (2) spares the thumb. The degloving usually extends up to the wrist crease or on to the forearm. The planning of the incision in the abdominal wall depends on the type of degloving.
   - The hand is going to be buried in the abdominal wall. So the hand is first placed over the abdomen to plan the area of the abdominal wall which is going to be used for the reconstruction (Fig. 2.8.1).
   - If the thumb is spared from the degloving, the infraumbilical segment of the abdomen is enough. But if the thumb is also degloved, the supraumbilical segment of the abdominal wall will also be required.
   - The method of planning consists of the incision and the area for creating a pocket. The incision length will be decided by the length of the skin on the proximal edge of the defect.
   - The incision is made through the skin and subcutaneous tissues. It is not necessary to make the incision down to the fascia.
8. The abdominal pocket must be created carefully (Fig. 2.8.2) with blunt dissection to avoid injuring the multiple paraumbilical perforators.
9. The degloved hand can be inserted off and on to ensure a comfortable lie within its pocket.
10. Once the pocket created is of adequate size, and the hand lies comfortably in the pocket, the skin can be sutured at the proximal edge.
11. This position must be maintained for a period of 3 weeks.

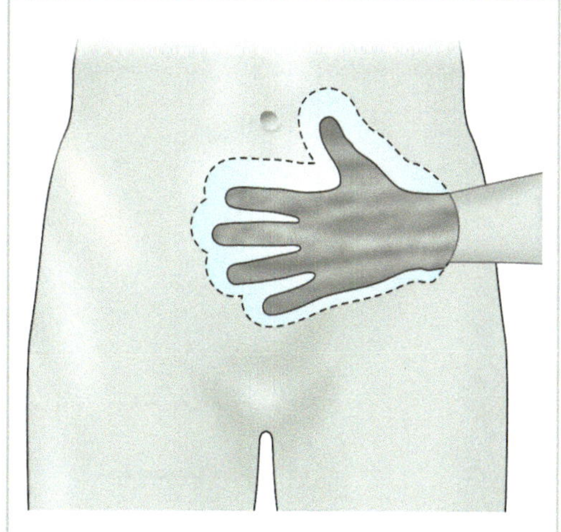

Fig. 2.8.1 Marking the area on the abdomen which is to be used for the buried flap

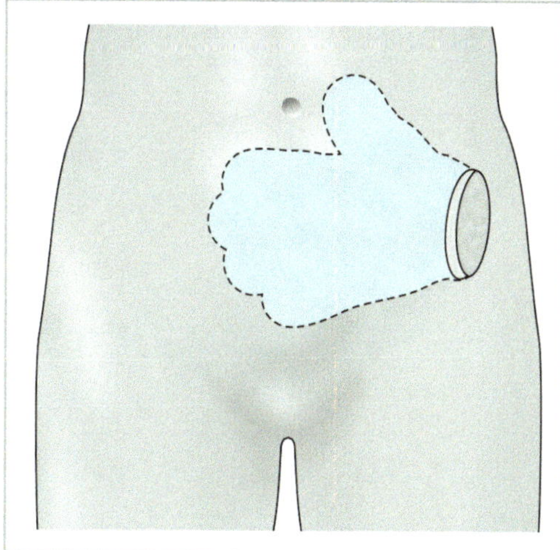

Fig. 2.8.2 Showing the abdominal pocket created for burying the degloved hand

Postoperative Protocol after Flap Stage I

- Admission in the ward
- The affected hand should be kept elevated
- Patient can take normal diet immediately if the procedure was under regional block or after complete recovery if under general anesthesia.
- Clinical monitoring of the flap once every 6 hours.
- Analgesics and antibiotics for 5 days.
- Sedation sos for 1 day.
- Inspection of the dressing after 48 hours.
- Removal of sutures on the 10th postoperative day.

The further procedure will depend on whether partial Crane technique or full Crane technique is planned:

Partial Crane technique: Here, at the end of 2 weeks, a delay procedure is planned.

12. This surgery can be done under local anesthesia, or regional block anesthesia.
13. The outline of the hand that has been buried in the abdominal wall is palpated carefully. A marking is made about 2 to 3 cm beyond the margins of the palpated hand and thumb. All the fingers are taken a single unit. When marking around the thumb, the proximity to the umbilicus must be considered. It is ideal to spare the umbilicus and plan the markings around the umbilicus. Hence the marking will now be as shown in the diagram (Fig. 2.8.3). This marking will be the planned incision for the delay procedure.
14. An incision is made along the markings, through the skin and subcutaneous tissues. Hemostasis is achieved and the wound is sutured with 3.0 polyamide suture.
15. A sterile dressing is done.
16. *Division of the flap:* This is done at the end of 3 weeks—1 week after the delay procedure was done.
17. This surgery is done under regional block anesthesia with supraclavicular block anesthesia or general anesthesia.
18. The same incision is made as was used for the delay procedure. First the sutures of the delay procedure are removed and a wash given with povidone-iodine solution.
19. The incision is made down to the fascia and the hand is removed along with the overlying abdominal skin flap which covers the dorsum of the hand (Fig. 2.8.4).
20. The bed will now consist of the fascia of the abdominal wall. Now the hand is examined. Hemostasis is achieved. Both the raw area in the abdominal wall (Fig. 2.8.5) and the palmar surface of the hand (Fig. 2.8.6) are covered with skin graft harvested from the thigh.

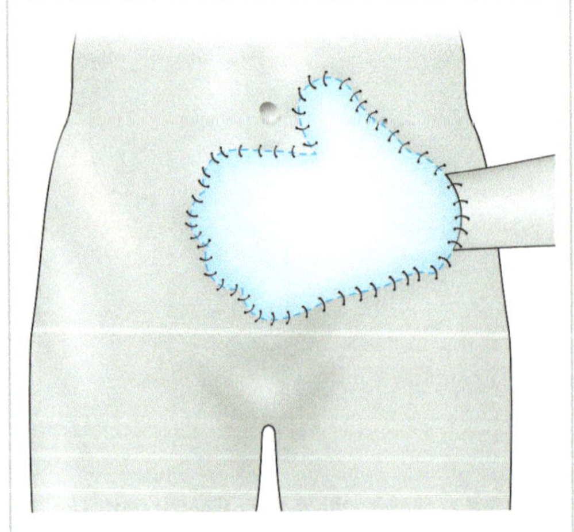

Fig. 2.8.3 Delay of the flap

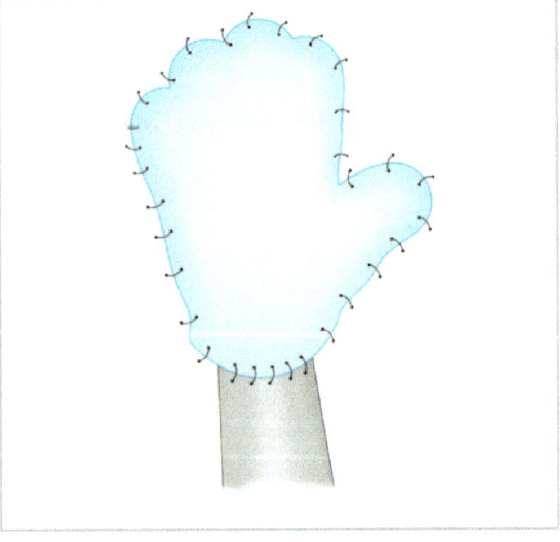

Fig. 2.8.4 Dorsal side of reconstructed hand

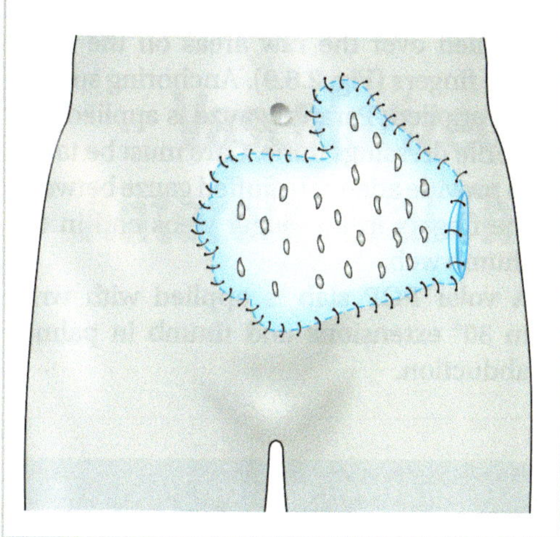

Fig. 2.8.5 Donor site with skin graft

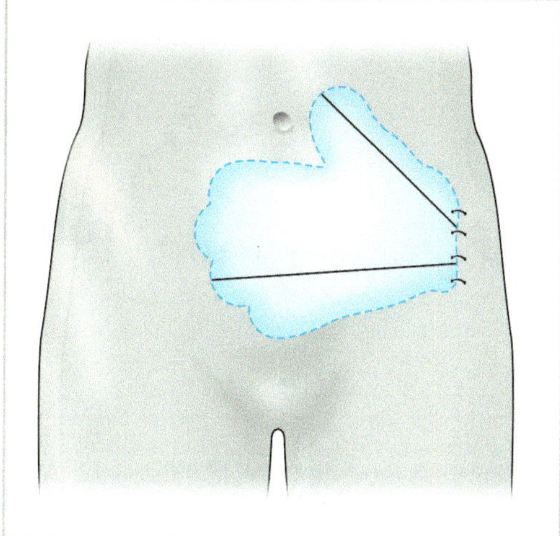

Fig. 2.8.7 Marking of incisions to explant the buried hand

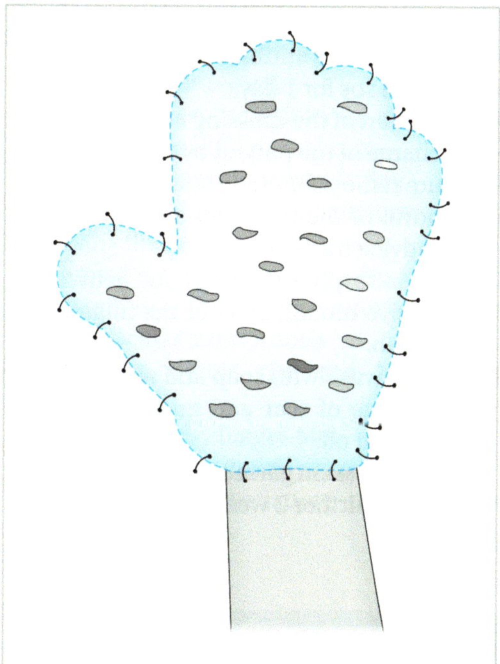

Fig. 2.8.6 Volar view of the reconstructed hand

21. Anchoring sutures are applied with 3.0 polyamide sutures and sterile dressings are applied after applying paraffin gauze.
22. On the hand, a volar plaster of Paris (POP) slab must be applied with the wrist in 30° extension, taking care to place adequate padding in the thumb web. The thumb must be kept in a position of palmar abduction.
    Full Crane technique: When this technique has been planned, flap division is planned at the end of 3 weeks.
23. The anesthesia required for the procedure of flap division is general anesthesia or a regional block with a supraclavicular block anesthesia.
24. The abdominal wall and the involved upper limb is prepared and draped.
25. Incisions are made over the palpated hand which has been buried in the abdominal wall (Fig. 2.8.7).
26. The skin flaps are raised on the abdominal wall superficial to the hand. In this way, the entire buried hand is exposed, retaining a coating of soft tissues acquired from the abdominal wall.
27. The hand is now removed from its bed. The soft tissue cover can also be noticed on the palmar aspect.
28. Hemostasis is achieved on the abdominal wall. The wounds are closed primarily (Fig. 2.8.8) after keeping drainage tubes and sterile dressings are applied.
29. Now the hand wound is thoroughly washed with a solution of povidone-iodine, hydrogen peroxide and saline.

pedicle. Now the pedicle is ready. Apply pledgets of gauze soaked in 1 percent xylocaine solution over the vessels.

11. Now, draw an imaginary line between the points "A" and the distal point of the musculocutaneous perforator. This imaginary line represents the approximate course of the perforator through the vastus lateralis muscle. Now make an incision about 1 cm *caudal* to this imaginary line and parallel to it. This incision will go down to the muscle after dividing the deep fascia. Incise the muscle also carefully, cauterizing the three to four vascular branches from our perforator. Similarly, draw an imaginary line between the point "B" and the distal point of the septocutaneous perforator. This imaginary line represents the approximate course of the perforator through the intermuscular septum. Now make an incision about 1 cm *cephalad* to this imaginary line and parallel to it. This incision goes through the septum and divides it.
12. Draw an imaginary line connecting the points "A" and "B". This represents the *vascular hilum* of the flap. On the undersurface of the flap that we have so far raised, we can see the deep fascia as a dense white layer. Make a marking on this layer, 1 cm medial to the line "AB". So the only fascia we require in our flap is the fascia required to protect the vascular hilum. Continue this line distally and proximally for 2 cm. Make the incisions on the markings.

> During the entire procedure of dissection of the pedicle, the vessels must be constantly bathed with 1 percent solution of xylocaine. This will prevent spasm of the vessels.

13. Replace the flap back. Make the remaining incisions of the proximal, lateral and distal borders of the flap. The flap should be raised from these sides superficial to the deep fascia. There will be a number of small perforators to the skin. These should be cauterized while raising the flap. Stop the dissection when the point of the vascular hilum is reached. Make an incision on the deep fascia about 1 cm lateral to the vascular hilum. So now the entire hilum is protected by fascia. With gentle lateral retraction of the flap, the remaining muscle fibers are separated, thus freeing the entire pedicle.
14. The flap is replaced back and two to three anchoring sutures are placed with 3.0 ethilon to the medial skin edge to prevent the flap from shearing. Bleeding is checked from the edges of the flap. A small streak is made on the distal most portion of the skin flap to confirm the slow and steady ooze of bright-red blood.
15. *Flap thinning:* The anchoring suture should be removed and the flap freed. It should be turned over and the flap thinned with heavy curved scissors passed parallel to the surface of the skin. The area around the vascular hilum should not be thinned.
16. The pedicle should be divided only after the vessels have been dissected and kept ready on the hand.
17. *Division of the pedicle:* Usually, there are two veins and one artery at the point of origin of the vessels from the descending branch of the lateral circumflex vessels. The artery and veins should be dissected free. Soft clamps should be applied over the artery and veins. The proximal ends of the artery and veins should be ligated with 3.0 vicryl. The vessels should be divided and the time noted. The flap should be placed on a moist abdominal pad with the raw area facing upward and taken to the recipient site for vascular anastomosis.
18. *Management of the donor site:* After securing hemostasis, the secondary defect should be narrowed with 3.0 vicryl and the proximal end closed primarily with 3.0 ethilon. There will be a residual raw area if the flap has been a big one. This should be covered with a split skin graft harvested

from the posterior aspect of the same thigh. The graft should be applied over the raw area and tie over sutures applied with 3.0 ethilon. Sterile dressings should be applied and elastocrépe bandage applied over it.

Vascular Anastomosis

19. The flap is brought to the hand defect. First the flap is held up and the pedicle allowed hanging down. This step will make sure that there is no inadvertent twisting of the vascular pedicle. The flap is then placed over the defect with the correct orientation and the end of the pedicle should be placed over the recipient vessels. A few sutures should be applied to inset the flap.
20. The recipient vessels should be divided, blood flow checked from the divided artery and approximator clamps applied. The soft clamps must be released from the donor vessels. Vascular anastomosis should be done. (The technique of vascular anastomosis is beyond the scope of this manual).

SECTION

3

Other Post-traumatic Sequelae on the Skin

Adherent Scars and Contractures

10

Introduction

Even if there are no raw areas on the upper limb, the condition of the skin is the most important point to be assessed. There are certain features to be examined and evaluated before the deeper structures can be assessed.

The nature of the skin on the upper limb may be consisted of any one of the following types:

- Soft and supple skin
- No scars but indurated skin
- Linear scars following healing by primary intention
- Linear scars following healing by secondary intention
- Hypertrophic scars
- Pigmented scars
- Depigmented scars
- Atrophic scars
- Adherent scars
- Contracted scars.

Examination of the Scar

- *The site of the scar:* It gives an idea about the probable injury to the underlying tissues. For example, if there is a scar on the flexor aspect of the forearm, it indicates possible injury to the flexor tendons and median and ulnar nerves.
- *The length of the scar:* It will also give an idea about the possible structures injured. A scar on the flexor aspect of the forearm that is limited to the ulnar side is most likely to have involved only the ulnar side structures such as the ulnar nerve and the flexors of the ring and little fingers.
- *The width of the scar:* A scar that has healed by primary intention is usually thin, while a scar that has healed by secondary intention is wider.
- *Shape of the scar:* In some situations the shape of the scar will give a clue about the cause. For example, if the patient has made an attempt to camouflage a tattoo on the forearm with chemicals, the pattern of the burn and the site of the burn will point toward a self-inflicted injury.
- *The color of the scar:* Some scars are hyperpigmented, especially the scars that have been caused by very superficial flame burns that have not been adequately protected during the healing phase. Scars that have formed from healing of superficial abrasions also tend to behave in the same way. The other types of scars that are hyperpigmented are grafted skin scars, which become hyperpigmented with time.
- *The thickness of the scar:* This will indicate the nature of the lesion that caused the scar. If the scar is wide and hypertrophic, it may have been caused by secondary healing of a wound, or if it is broad and hypertrophic, it might have been caused by flame burns.
- *The relationship of the scar to the underlying tissues:* This is an indicator of the pliability

of the skin. Even when there is no scar, the skin may appear edematous and may not move passively over the underlying tissues when it is indurated. Sometimes grafted skin also becomes adherent to the underlying tissues.

- *Contracture bands:* May also develop following trauma. The essential management of such contractures is similar to the management of contractures following burns. However, the treatment of post-traumatic contractures does not end with the management of the contracture as in burns. The underlying problem must also be dealt with accordingly.

There are certain problems caused by scars:

- Functional problems
  - Hypertrophic scars can cause functional problems like contractures and limitation of movements on the upper limb.
  - Contractures on the skin can also cause deformities and hence functional deficit.
- Problems in later reconstruction
  - When scars are thin and atrophic, underlying problems of structures like tendon or bone cannot be accessed by incisions over this type of skin as wound healing may be poor. Similarly, adherent scars and hypertrophic scars have also to be corrected before any reconstructive surgery can be planned on the underlying tissues.
- Cosmetic problems
  - Are also important, because hands are exposed parts of the body and unacceptable scars on these areas may damage the body image.

Management Protocol

The set of management protocol is given in Table 3.10.1.

Table 3.10.1 Management protocol

Nature of skin or scar	*Management*
Edematous skin	Hand elevation Anti-inflammatory drugs
Indurated skin	Compression garments Scar massage
Linear scar with no tissue problem	Compression
Linear scar with underlying tissue problem requiring	Excision of scar during tissue reconstruction
Contracture skin	Release contracture as in chapter on contractures
Hypertrophic scar with no functional deficit	Compression If no response after 6 months—plan for excision and grafting
Hypertrophic scar with functional deficit Thin atrophic scar Adherent scar	Excision and flap cover (flap cover planned according to area as in previous segment)
Depigmented scar	Excision and skin grafting

SECTION

4

Tendon Reconstruction

Tendon Reconstruction—Assessment

11

Introduction

When a patient presents at the outpatient department with a tendon injury, reconstruction must be planned with the following aims:

- To evaluate which tendons have been injured
- To evaluate the plan of reconstruction.

The following points should be noted:

- *History:* The nature of injury and the duration of injury
  - Nature of injury
    - If the injury has been a blunt injury with a forceful extension of a finger or a forceful flexion of a finger against resistance, there is most probably a tendon avulsion.
    - If the injury was by a penetration injury, most probably, a single tendon has been injured, but other injuries like nerve injuries should be ruled out.
    - If the injury was by a sharp instrument, it is likely that many tendons are injured along with nerves. Hence, a thorough assessment is necessary.
    - If the injury was by a heavy object, leading to skin loss, the tendons injured also have segmental loss, which must be taken into account during assessment.
    - If the injury was by avulsion, it is most likely that the entire tendon and muscle have been lost and this will require special attention in planning the treatment.
- *Duration of injury:* Apart from primary management of tendon injuries which have not been dealt with in this manual, patients may present later and require treatment:
  - *Less than 10 days:* In such a situation, the tendon repair can be done at the end of 10 days when the sutures have been removed and the wound is dry.
  - *Between 10 days and 3 weeks:* If the patient has presented during this period, it is ideal not to plan for any surgical management immediately, but to wait till 3 weeks are over after the injury. This is because the tissues are in the inflammatory phase and any surgical management will result in more scar formation and subsequently, more adhesions between the tendons and other tissues. Moreover, when the patient is taken up for surgery by the end of 3 weeks, the tendons are so retracted that it may be impossible to do primary repair of the tendons. In such situations, a tendon grafting is ideal for all the flexor tendons and extensor tendons of the fingers except the flexor pollicis longus (FPL) tendon and the extensor pollicis longus (EPL) tendon of the thumb. If there is a segmental loss of these two tendons or the proximal ends have retracted, it is ideal to do a tendon transfer for these tendons, rather than a tendon

grafting. However, this waiting period can be utilized to mobilize the fingers and hand to keep the joints supple and to strengthen muscles.
  - *More than 1 year after injury:* Sometimes, patients turn-up even a year after the injury, to have reconstruction done. In such patients, since primary repair of the tendons will not be possible, tendon grafting will have to be done. However, the bulk of the muscle should be assessed before planning the tendon graft. This is because the muscle might have undergone atrophy by this time, and may not be able to move the tendon after grafting. Hence, in such situations, a tendon transfer is better suited for such patients.
- The nature of the skin over the affected area:
  - If there has been an avulsion of the tendon as in case of flexor digitorum profundus (FDP) avulsion, the skin will grossly appear normal, but tell-tale signs of bruising and contusion can be made out in the early few days after injury.
  - If there was a penetrating injury, a very small scar may be seen that may belie the magnitude of injury.
  - In case of an assault or an injury with a sharp instrument, the scar will indicate the structures that are most probably injured. This scar should be soft and supple before any surgical management is planned.
  - If there was a skin loss which has already been treated with a skin cover, this should also be noted. The quality of the skin cover is very important:
    - If the skin over the injured tendon is a skin graft, it is necessary to resurface this area with a skin flap before tendon surgery can be done. This is because the skin grafted area will not withstand incisions and wound healing will be poor.
    - If the skin over the area is a skin flap, which is thin and soft, surgery can be done for the tendons through this skin.
    - If the skin flap is bulky, it is ideal to do the first stage of thinning the flap and making it more cosmetically acceptable, before the stage of tendon reconstruction.
    - In long standing problems, the skin may have been contracted over the area of tendon injury as happens in cases of tendon injuries in children. In such situations, a contracture release is done before tendon reconstruction is attempted.
- The finger or fingers affected by the tendon injury should be noted.
- The status of the joints of the hand and of the affected fingers in particular must be noted. This assessment must include the active range of movement and the passive range of movement. This is particularly useful in patients who are presenting late for treatment, as the joints become stiff if regular physiotherapy has not been done.
- *Any concomitant injury:* It is important to look for other injuries which are likely to have happened along with the tendon injury.
  - *Nerve injury:* If this is the case, reconstruction of the nerve should also be planned when the tendon reconstruction is done.
  - *Bone injury:* If there has been a fracture along with the tendon damage at the time of injury, the bony status should be assessed.
    - *If good union:* No bony work is required.
    - *If fracture malunited but in acceptable position:* Tendon reconstruction can be carried out right away and it is not

Table 4.11.1 Clinical examination

Tendon tested	*Instructions for the patient*
Flexor digitorum profundus of the finger	Hold the middle phalangeal segment of the finger and ask the patient to flex the distal interphalangeal (DIP) joint
Flexor digitorum superficialis (FDS) of the finger-middle, ring and little	Place the palm flat on the table with the fingers straight. Place the examining hand on the fingers except the one that is being tested and restrain the fingers. Ask the patient to flex only the finger that is being tested
Flexor digitorum superficialis of index finger	Hold the DIP joint of index finger in hyperextension and ask patient to flex PIP joint
Flexor pollicis longus	Hold the proximal phalangeal segment of the thumb and ask the patient to flex the interphalangeal (IP) joint of the thumb
Extensor digitorum communis (EDC) of the fingers	Ask the patient to place the palm flat on the table. Ask the patient to lift-up the finger being tested
Extensor indicis proprius (EIP) of index finger	Ask the patient to make a fist. Now, ask the patient to lift and point the index finger
Extensor digiti minimi (EDM) of the little finger	Ask the patient to make a fist. Now, ask the patient to lift and point the little finger
Extensor pollicis longus (EPL)	Hold the proximal phalangeal segment of the thumb and ask the patient to extend the IP joint of the thumb
Palmaris longus	Oppose the tip of the thumb to the tip of the little finger and flex the wrist. The tendon can be palpated
Extensors of fingers	Make a fist and then extend the wrist
Flexors of the wrist	Make a fist and flex the wrist

Table 4.11.2 Diagnosis and management plan

Diagnosis	*Management plan*
Injury to flexor or extensor tendon less than 10 days duration	Delayed primary tendon repair
Injury to flexor or extensor tendon of the finger less than 3 months duration Or segmental loss of flexor or extensor tendon of the finger	Tendon grafting
Segmental loss of flexor tendon with injury to pulley system as evidenced by long duration (> 1 year) extensive scarring over the fingers	Staged flexor tendon reconstruction
Injury to flexor or extensor tendon of the thumb greater than 3 months duration Or segmental loss of flexor or extensor tendon of the thumb	Tendon transfer
Avulsion of the flexor tendon of the finger	Reattachment of the flexor tendon/flexor tendon grafting with pull-out suture
Repaired or reconstructed tendon with no active movement	Tendon transfer
Repaired or reconstructed tendon with less than full active movement, but full passive movement	Flexor tenolysis

essential to correct trivial malunion unless it interferes with function.

- *If malunion and not acceptable:* Osteotomy is required and refixation should be done in a first stage before tendon reconstruction can be taken up.
- If nonunion is present, this should be dealt with appropriately, and the stage of tendon reconstruction should be done later when the bone problem has been settled.

Clinical Examination

The details of clinical examinations has been given in Table 4.11.1:

Deciding on the Plan of Management

The diagnosis and management plan is explained in Table 4.11.2.

Repair of Avulsed Flexor Tendon

12

Introduction

The condition of an avulsed flexor tendon can present either at the emergency theater or in the outpatient clinic. Recognition of the condition is by the following features:

- History of blunt injury by a hyperextension of the finger—may occur after a fall on the hand, or by a forceful flexion of the finger when the finger is locked in extension—as in a sports injury when the finger is caught in the shirt of another player.
- Total inability to flex both interphalangeal (IP) joints of the finger, even though only the flexor profundus tendon is avulsed. This is because the retracted flexor tendon recedes in the pulley and may get caught in the chiasma of the flexor superficialis. Hence, the superficialis tendon may also get locked.
- Tell-tale signs of bruising on the finger on the volar aspect at the terminal phalanx level may be present.
- An X-ray may reveal the proximal end of the avulsed tendon, if there has been an associated fracture of the volar lip of the terminal phalanx, where the flexor profundus tendon is inserted.

The treatment of this condition consists of exploration and reattachment of the avulsed flexor tendon.

Presurgical Counseling

- This procedure will be done under axillary block anesthesia or general anesthesia (in children)
- The procedure consists of reattaching the avulsed tendon
- This procedure will take about 1½ to 2 hours to perform
- A dressing will be applied and a plaster of Paris (POP) slab will be applied at the end of surgery
- Admission will be necessary for a minimum period of 3 days
- Postoperatively, no movements of the fingers should be attempted. If it is done, the sutured tendon may rupture
- Postoperatively, the POP slab will be continued for a period of 3 weeks. After this period, physiotherapy will be started and this should be done for another 5 weeks
- In some instances, even if the movements of the finger improve, further surgery may be required to release the scars that may form
- The general complications of anesthetic infiltration like hypersensitivity may occur in spite of test dose application. This complication will cause dryness of mouth and apprehension, which can be corrected immediately.

Surgical Steps

1. First, the hand is prepared for surgery as described in Appendix I.
2. Marking the incisions:
   - First, make a marking on the neutral line of the noncontact surface of the finger from the web region to the distal interphalangeal (DIP) joint crease. This means that the incision should be made on the ulnar side for the index, middle and ring finger and the radial side for the little finger.
   - From the DIP joint crease level, extend the incision distally across the volar aspect of the terminal phalangeal segment (pulp region) in an oblique manner to reach the opposite side of the finger near the tip.
   - From the point on the web region, extend the incision proximally in an oblique manner to reach the distal palmar crease. This marking may have to be extended proximally later, but this is the preliminary marking for the exploration of the flexor tendon of the finger and palm.
3. Now, the tourniquet is raised and the incisions are made. Make the incisions down to the subcutaneous tissue. On the neutral line segment and the terminal phalanx region, take care to avoid injuring the digital neurovascular bundle. Raise the entire skin and soft tissues of the volar aspect of the finger. Thus, the digital neurovascular bundle on the noncontact surface of the finger will be retained on the finger and the flap will be raised superficial to it. The flap continues to be raised superficial to the fibrous flexor sheath. This dissection stops when the digital neurovascular bundle of the opposite side of the finger comes into view.
4. Now, raise the palmar portion of the flap along with the fat pad (superficial to the palmar aponeurosis). The noncontact side neurovascular bundle and the flexor tendon sheath will be visible on the bed.
5. Anchor the raised skin flaps with 3.0 Ethilon after applying gentle traction on the skin flaps to afford maximal exposure of the entire flexor tendon sheath of the finger.
6. Now, the entire flexor sheath is exposed. Examine the sheath to look for signs of the proximal end of the avulsed and retracted tendon.
7. Hematoma under the tendon sheath that is visible.
8. Swelling in the flexor sheath at the level of the proximal phalanx segment of the finger.
9. If the tendon end seems to be lying in the tunnel distal to the middle of the proximal phalangeal region (distal to A2 pulley), make a small incision about 1 cm long transversely across this site, and try to retrieve the avulsed tendon from this opening in the sheath. If this is difficult, a proximal extension of the incision of the tendon sheath can be made on one side, parallel to the underlying tendon.
10. If the tendon end seems to be lying in the tunnel in the level of A2 pulley, do not make any incision on the tendon sheath, as the A2 pulley is very important for function and flexor tendon movement, and any scarring in this area will compromise movement. So, go proximal to the A1 pulley which is seen in the palm level. If it is possible, retrieve the tendon proximally from the A1 pulley level. If this is not possible, as happens when there is a segment of bone attached to the end of the avulsed tendon, make an incision over the tendon sheath as described in step 9.
11. Now, dissect the terminal segment of the flexor tendon sheath. Make an incision on one side of the tendon sheath at this level and reflect the flap of the sheath to expose the point of insertion of the flexor profundus tendon into the base of the terminal phalanx. This place will be empty due to the avulsed tendon. Identify the volar aspect of the base of the terminal phalanx and debride this area. There must

be a small raw area of the bone into which the tendon is going to be reattached.

12. Take a polyethylene tube—a scalp vein set tube with the needle end cut-off (retain this needle end for use later). Thread the free end of the tube into the tendon sheath from the distal end. Try to reach the point where the opening has been made in the tendon sheath to retrieve the proximal end. Deliver the free end of the tube in this point. Attach the avulsed end of the flexor tendon to the polyethylene tube with 3.0 polypropylenes suture using horizontal suture technique (Fig. 4.12.1).
13. Now, gently pull on the distal end of the polyethylene tube to railroad the tendon through the remaining segment of the intact flexor sheath, to the point of insertion at the terminal phalanx.
14. Now, the entire flexor tendon has been repositioned in the flexor sheath, and the reattachment must be done. Take a stitch in the free end of the tendon with 3.0 polypropylenes using Kessler Mason technique, and keep it ready. Cut-off the needle of the suture material and leave both ends of the suture material long. It does not matter if there is a small segment of bone in this, the suturing of the tendon will be enough to jam the bone segment into the raw area that has been created in the volar aspect of the terminal phalanx.

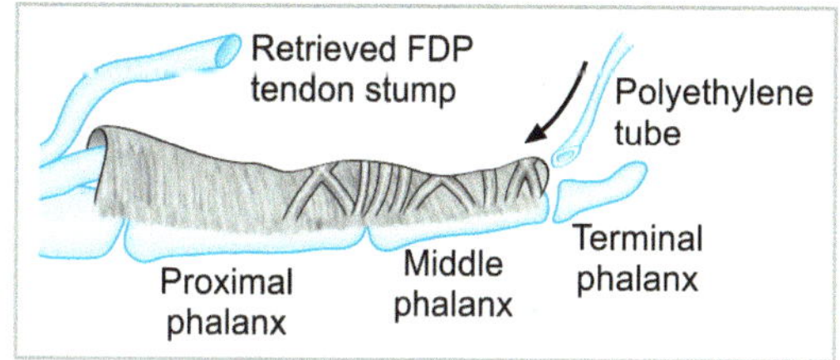

Fig. 4.12.1 Retrieving the proximal retracted flexor digitorum profundus (FDP) tendon

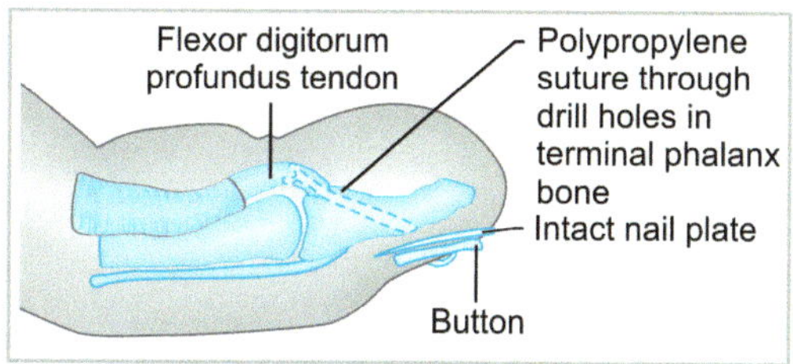

Fig. 4.12.2 Attaching the FDP tendon to the bone

15. Make two drill holes from the volar aspect of the base of the terminal phalanx to exit on the nail plate (Fig. 4.12.2). The two holes must be at a distance of a minimum of 2 to 3 mm. Thread the two free ends of the suture material that are on the end of the tendon through the two drill holes, to exit on the nail plate. If this is difficult, it can be done by passing an 18G needle from the nail plate end and then threading the suture material ends through the needle bore.
16. Now, the tendon has been replaced at its insertion and the two free ends of the suture material are exiting through the holes on the nail plate. Take the needle end of the scalp vein set that had been cut-off earlier. It has two polyethylene wings. Cut one of these wings, make two holes in it about 2 to 3 mm apart with an 18G needle. Thread the two free ends of the suture material through these holes, hold the "button" close to the nail plate and tie the suture securely with surgical knots.
17. Apply gentle compression with moist gauze and padding over the wound. Release the tourniquet. Hold the hand in an elevated position for a period of 4 to 5 minutes. Rest the hand on the table and secure hemostasis. The finger will now be seen in its attitude of normal cascade. Repair the wound made on the flexor tendon sheath with 5.0 polypropylenes using horizontal mattress suture, with the knots lying outside the sheath.
18. Suture the skin with 4.0 Ethilon after keeping Segmüller drains.

> It is important to get good hemostasis before suturing the skin. Hematomas are bad in any surgery and more so in this type of tendon surgery because, along with problems in wound healing, there is a compromise in function of the tendon.

19. Apply sterile dressings, and apply a dorsal below elbow POP slab, extending till the tips of the fingers, with the wrist in neutral position, metacarpophalangeal (MCP) joints of the fingers in 90° position and the IP joints straight.

Postoperative Protocol

The postoperative follow-up protocol of this surgery is very important.

- Admission in the ward
- The affected hand should be kept elevated
- Patient can take normal diet immediately if the procedure was under regional block or after complete recovery if under general anesthesia
- Inspection of the suture line after 48 hours without disturbing the position of the POP slab
- Discharge of the patient by third day
- Suture removal on the 10th day. Do not remove the dorsal button suture
- Patient to retain the POP slab
- Removal of the POP slab on the 21st day and advise the following:
  - Refer to physiotherapy for active mobilization of the fingers
  - Daily wash with soap and water
  - Massage of scar and grafted skin with coconut oil
- Review the patient after another 1 week and remove the dorsal button suture. Advise the patient to continue:
  - Active mobilization of the fingers
  - Daily wash with soap and water
  - Massage of scar and grafted skin with coconut oil
- Review the patient again after another 2 weeks (total of 6 weeks after surgery), assess the movements and advise
  - Passive mobilization and passive stretching of the finger
  - To apply straightening splint for the finger at night and to continue active and passive mobilization of the fingers during the day. This should be done for 2 weeks.

Flexor Tendon Grafting

13

Introduction

The most common indications for flexor tendon grafting are:

- Neglected injuries of flexor tendons presenting after a period of 3 weeks after injury (especially at Zone II level).
- Segmental loss of flexor tendons due to trauma, electrical burns.

Flexor tendon grafting can be done only in situations where the native muscle of the particular tendon is intact. For example, if there is a segmental loss of flexor tendon in the fingers, and another burn on the forearm in which all the muscles have been lost, a flexor tendon graft cannot be done. In such situations, tendon transfers are preferable from the tendons of healthy muscles.

Considering the example of a flexor tendon graft planned for a finger flexor, it can be planned to use the flexor superficialis tendon as a graft for the flexor digitorum profundus (FDP). Hence, only the FDP tendon is going to be reconstructed.

If the flexor digitorum superficialis (FDS) tendon is not available, the palmaris longus tendon can be harvested and used as a tendon graft.

Presurgical Counseling

- This procedure will be done under axillary block anesthesia or general anesthesia (in children)
- The procedure consists of harvesting a tendon graft from either the forearm (in case of one or two fingers) and from the thigh (in case of more than two fingers)
- This procedure will take about 2½ to 3 hours to perform or depends on the number of fingers involved
- A dressing will be applied and a plaster of Paris (POP) slab will be applied at the end of surgery
- Admission will be necessary for a minimum period of 3 days
- Postoperatively, no movements of the fingers should be attempted. If it is done, the sutured tendons may rupture
- Postoperatively, the POP slab will be continued for a period of 3 weeks. After this period, physiotherapy will be started and this should be done for another 3 weeks
- In some instances, even if the movements of the finger improve, further surgery may be required to release the scars that may form
- The general complications of anesthetic infiltration like hypersensitivity may occur in spite of test dose application. This complication will cause dryness of mouth and apprehension, which can be corrected immediately.

Surgical Steps

1. First, the hand is prepared for surgery as described in Appendix I.

aspect of the ulnar half of the forearm, about 3 cm proximal to the wrist crease. The incision is made through the skin and subcutaneous tissues, to expose the flexor tendons of the fingers
- The tendon of the FDS to the involved finger is identified by applying traction on the tendons and noting the movements
- The cut end of the FDS tendon which has already been identified and dissected in the palm is pulled and cut
- It is retrieved from the wrist wound by pulling on the FDS tendon
- Another transverse incision 3.0 cm is made about 6 to 7 cm more proximally on the forearm after applying traction on the cut end of the tendon and palpating the taut tendon under the skin
- The FDS is retrieved through this wound, and divided to close to the musculotendinous junction
- The tendon is placed in a cup of normal saline till its use.

- *Harvesting the Palmaris longus tendon as a graft*: It has been described in Appendix (VII)
- *Harvesting the fascia lata graft:* It is described in Appendix (VIII).

11. *Fixing the tendon graft*:
    - *Distal tendon anastomosis:* Once the tendon graft has been harvested, the tendon grafting can be done. First the distal tendon anastomosis is done. Before that, the tunnel for the tendon graft to be routed is made ready
    - Take a polyethylene tube—a scalp vein set tube with the needle end cut-off. Thread the free end of the tube into the tendon sheath from the distal end. Retrieve the proximal end of the tube in the palm, proximal to the flexor tendon sheath. Deliver the free end of the tube in this point. Attach the distal end of the tendon graft to the polyethylene tube with 3.0 polypropylenes suture using horizontal suture technique
    - Now, gently pull on the distal end of the polyethylene tube to railroad the tendon through the entire length of the flexor sheath, to the point of distal tendon edge at the terminal phalanx
    - Now, the entire flexor tendon graft has been repositioned in the flexor sheath
    - The distal end of the tendon graft is attached to the distal cut end of the FDP tendon by one of these two methods:
        a. If the size of the cut end of the tendon graft is equal to the size of the distal FDP tendon, the suturing is done with 3.0 polypropylenes using modified Kessler Mason Allen suture (Fig. 4.13.2)
        b. If the size of the cut end of the tendon graft is smaller than the distal cut end of the FDP tendon, the following technique is used. The distal FDP tendon is split into two longitudinally for about 1 cm. The distal end of the tendon graft is inserted in between the two parts. A stitch is taken with 3.0 polypropylenes from the side, through one part of the FDP tendon, then through the tendon graft, and again through the second part of the FDP tendon. This stitch is then turned back through the same layers in reverse and the knot is tied (Fig. 4.13.3) Another stitch of the same type can be applied distal to the first,

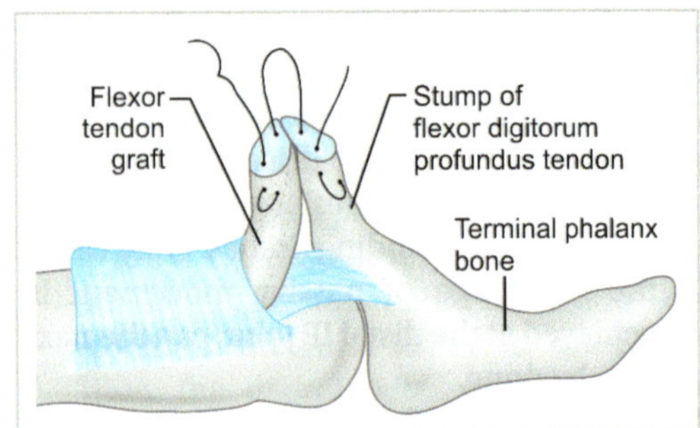

Fig. 4.13.2 Method of distal tendon repair of equal size

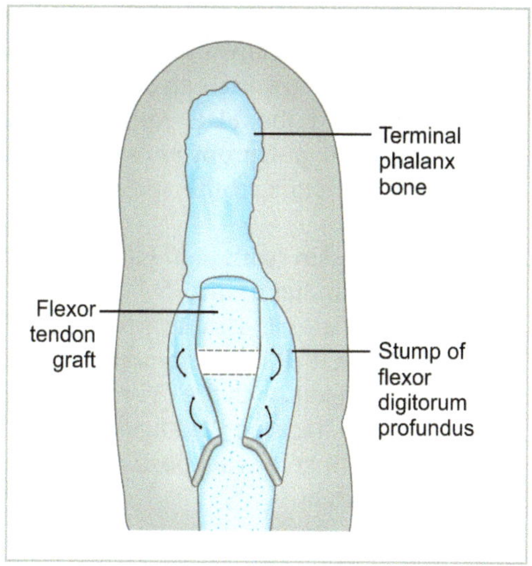

Fig. 4.13.3 Method of tendon repair if tendon graft is smaller

to reinforce the distal attachment. This suturing should be secured. It should be remembered that the common cause of tendon dehiscence occurs at the distal anastomosis

- The extralength of the tendon graft should be excised and stored in saline as mentioned above, and can be used as material for pulley reconstruction
- Once the distal suturing is over, the free end of the tendon graft that is at the palm level should be gently pulled and the movement pattern of the finger at the IP joints noted. The finger-tip should touch the palm. If this does not happen, or, the movement is not satisfactory, the pulley system should be examined
- If there is a deficit at the A2 or A4 pulleys, they should be reconstructed
- *Pulley reconstruction:* The excess tendon graft should be applied over the area where the pulley is to be reconstructed. One end should be sutured to the remnant of the original pulley with 5.0 polypropylenes using horizontal suture technique with the knot coming outside. The tendon graft is then laid transversely over the tendon graft and sutured to the other side remnant of the pulley with 5.0 polypropylenes using horizontal suture technique with the knot coming outside. Care should be taken that the reconstructed pulley is not so tight as to prevent the flexor tendon from moving, nor so loose that the tendon bowstrings on moving
- Apply gentle compression with moist gauze and padding over the wound. Release the tourniquet. Hold the hand in an elevated position for a period of 4 to 5 minutes. Rest the hand on the table and secure hemostasis. Now, the skin wound on the finger should be sutured with 4.0 Ethilon. The passive movement of the finger on pulling on the free end of the tendon graft, should again be confirmed

> It is important to get good hemostasis before suturing the skin. Hematomas are bad in any surgery and more so in this type of tendon surgery because, along with problems in wound healing, there is a compromise in function of the tendon.

12. *Proximal tendon anastomosis:* The proximal end of the tendon graft is now sutured to the cut end of the FDP tendon which has been dissected and kept ready (step 9). The important consideration in this step is the adjustment of tension in the tendon graft:
    - Pull the cut end of the FDP tendon. It should glide freely forward and backward. If it does not do so, further mobilization should be done until it does so. Pull the tendon to the maximum. Make a mark on the tendon at the point where it just becomes visible in the wound. Mark this point as "A". Now, relax the tendon and it will glide back into the forearm for a certain distance. Now, mark the point where the tendon just becomes visible at the edge of the wound. Mark this point as "B". So, the distance "AB" is the amplitude of movement of the

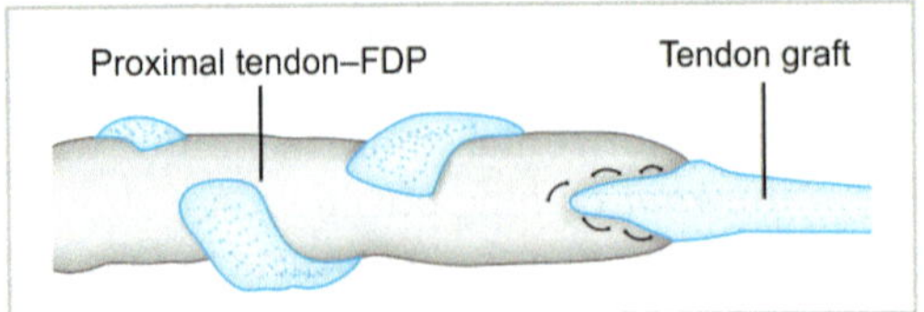

Fig. 4.13.4 Pulvertaft technique of tendon suturing

FDP tendon. Mark the midpoint of the distance "AB" and mark this point as "C". Hold the tendon in such a way that the point "C" is just visible at the edge of the wound. This should be the position of the FDP while it is being sutured to the tendon graft, with the finger in a position of normal cascade.

- Pull the free end of the tendon graft so that the finger is held in a position of the cascade of the finger. Now, freshen the two ends of the tendons and repair them in one of the following methods:
  - If the size of the cut end of the tendon graft is equal to the size of the cut end of FDP, the suturing is done with 3.0 polypropylenes using modified Kessler Mason Allen suture
  - If the size of the cut end of the tendon graft is smaller than the distal cut end of the FDP tendon, the Pulvertaft technique (Fig. 4.13.4) is used
  - Hold the FDP tendon taut with a hemostat applied on the end and pulling distally
  - About 1 cm proximal to the end of the tendon, make a cut in a volar to dorsal direction with a number 11 blade, with just enough length to allow the tendon graft through. Pull the tendon graft through and adjust the tension so that the finger lies in the normal cascade. Apply a suture with 3.0 polypropylenes using horizontal mattress suture
  - About 1 cm proximal to the first cut, make another cut with number 11 blade, from a radial to ulnar direction. Thread the free end of the tendon graft through this opening also and suture with 3.0 polypropylenes using horizontal mattress suture
  - Trim the excess length of the tendon graft and the FDP. Apply sutures with 4.0 polypropylenes to attach the cut ends to the surface of the tendon.

13. Suture the skin with 4.0 Ethilon after keeping Segmüller drains.
14. Apply sterile dressings, and apply a dorsal below elbow POP slab, extending till the tips of the fingers, with the wrist in neutral position, metacarpophalangeal (MCP) joints of the fingers in 90° position and the IP joints straight.

Postoperative Protocol

The postoperative follow-up protocol of this surgery is very important.

- Admission in the ward
- The affected hand should be kept elevated
- Patient can take normal diet immediately if the procedure was under regional block or after complete recovery if under general anesthesia
- Inspection of the suture line after 48 hours without disturbing the position of the POP slab
- Discharge of the patient by third day
- Suture removal on the 10th day
- Patient to retain the POP slab
- Removals of the POP slab on the 21st day and advise the following:
  - Refer to physiotherapy for active mobilization of the fingers
  - Daily wash with soap and water
  - Massage of scar and grafted skin with coconut oil
- Review the patient again after another 2 weeks (total of 6 weeks after surgery), assess the movements and advice passive mobilization and passive stretching of the finger
- To apply straightening splint for the finger at night and to continue active and passive mobilization of the fingers during the day. This should be done for 2 weeks.

Staged Flexor Tendon Reconstruction

14

Introduction

In some cases where a tendon graft is required, the procedure should not be done as described in the previous chapter in a single stage. It should be done in a staged procedure consisting of two stages. This is usually prescribed when the duration is more than a year, or there are multiple scars on the involved fingers.

Presurgical Counseling

This procedure will consist of two stages. Both stages will be done under axillary block anesthesia or general anesthesia:

Stage I

- The first stage consists of inserting the silastic implant in the finger.
- This procedure will take about 1½ to 2 hours to perform.
- A dressing will be applied and a plaster of Paris (POP) slab will be applied at the end of surgery.
- Admission will be necessary for a minimum period of 3 days.
- Postoperatively, no movements of the fingers should be attempted. If it is done, the sutured tendons may rupture.
- Postoperatively, the POP slab will be continued for a period of 3 weeks. After this period, physiotherapy will be started and this should be done for another 3 weeks.
- Only after 3 months, the next stage will be done.
- In some rare instances, the implant may extrude. In this situation, the procedure will have to be redone with a new implant.
- The general complications of anesthetic infiltration like hypersensitivity may occur in spite of test dose application. This complication will cause dryness of mouth and apprehension, which can be corrected immediately.

Stage II

- The procedure consists of harvesting a tendon graft from either the forearm (in case of one or two fingers) and from the thigh (in case of more than two fingers).
- This procedure will take about 1½ to 2 hours to perform.
- A dressing will be applied and a POP slab will be applied at the end of surgery.
- Admission will be necessary for a minimum period of 3 days.
- Postoperatively, no movements of the fingers should be attempted. If it is done, the sutured tendons may rupture.
- Postoperatively, the POP slab will be continued for a period of 3 weeks. After this period, physiotherapy will be started and this should be done for another 3 weeks.
- In some instances, even if the movements of the finger improve, further surgery may be required to release the scars that may form.

- The general complications of anesthetic infiltration like hypersensitivity may occur in spite of test dose application. This complication will cause dryness of mouth and apprehension, which can be corrected immediately.

Surgical Steps

Stage I

- First the hand is prepared for surgery as described in Appendix I
- *Marking the incisions (Fig. 4.14.1):*
    - First make a marking "A" on the neutral line of the noncontact surface of the finger from the web region to the distal interphalangeal (DIP) joint crease. This means that the incision should be made on the ulnar side for the index, middle and ring fingers and the radial side for the little finger.
    - From the DIP joint crease level, extend the incision distally across the volar aspect of the terminal phalangeal segment (pulp region) in an oblique manner "B" to reach the opposite side of the finger near the tip.
    - From the point on the web region, extend the incision "C" proximally in an oblique manner to reach the distal palmar crease. This marking will have to be extended proximally to reach the proximal part of the hollow between the thenar and hypothenar eminences.
    - A longitudinal incision "D" on the forearm measuring about 5 to 6 cm, about 2 cm proximal to the wrist crease. This incision should be on the ulnar half of the distal forearm.

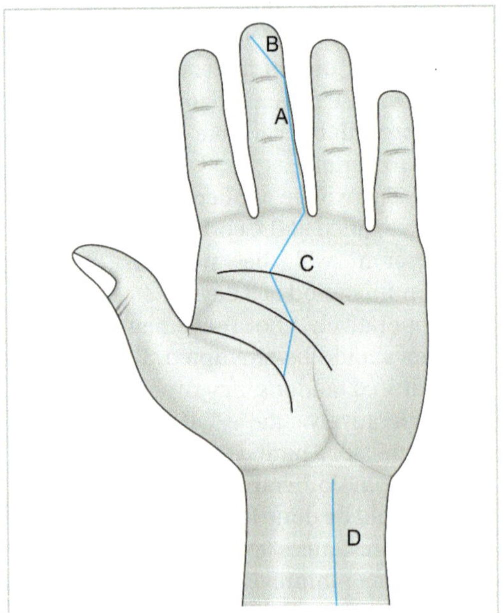

Fig. 4.14.1 Incision markings for stage I

- Make the incisions down to the subcutaneous tissue. On the neutral line segment and the terminal phalanx region, take care to avoid injuring the digital neurovascular bundle. Raise the entire skin and soft tissues of the volar aspect of the finger. Thus, the digital neurovascular bundle on the noncontact surface of the finger will be retained on the finger and the flap will be raised superficial to it. The flap continues to be raised superficial to the fibrous flexor sheath. This dissection stops when the digital neurovascular bundle of the opposite side of the finger comes into view.
- Now, raise the palmar portion of the flap along with the fat pad (superficial to the palmar aponeurosis). The noncontact side neurovascular bundle and the flexor tendon sheath will be visible on the bed.
- Anchor the raised skin flaps with 3.0 Ethilon after applying gentle traction on the skin flaps to afford maximal exposure of the entire flexor tendon sheath of the finger. Surgeons must look for any associated injury like that of a digital nerve which should be managed along with.
- *Distal tendon dissection*: The first step is to dissect the distal part of the tendon. This is the distal end of the flexor profundus tendon, as it is this tendon that surgeons are going to reconstruct. The distal part of the flexor tendon sheath is opened like a book, by making an incision on the

side of the flexor sheath at the level of the distal part of the middle phalanx and the terminal phalanx. This will expose the insertion of the flexor digitorum profundus (FDP) on the terminal phalanx.

- Usually, there will be about 2 to 2.5 cm of the tendon remaining inserted to bone. Only 2 cm should be retained for good attachment of the tendon graft. The longer this insertion is left, the less will be the leverage of the tendon, and hence, lesser will be the movement. Once the inserting tendon has been dissected, it should be pulled to see if full range of movement of the DIP joint is present. If there is a restriction of either the flexion or extension, further dissection must be done to free the adhesions with the volar plate and surrounding tissues. Only when the full range of passive movement is achieved at the DIP joint, can the next step be done.
- Now, consider the remaining segment of the flexor tendon sheath. This tunnel will usually be collapsed, and will contain:
    - The insertion of the flexor superficialis tendon (about 1–1.5 cm).
    - The proximal cut ends of the flexor superficialis and flexor profundus tendons may be present in the proximal part of the tunnel. Even if these tendons are present, they will be stuck by dense adhesions to the sides of the flexor tunnel.
    - The flexor sheath also will be weakened at some places and may not withstand dissection. The most important pulleys that must be preserved are the A2 pulley and the A4 pulley: that is, the pulley segment over the proximal part of the proximal phalanx region, and the pulley segment over the proximal part of the middle phalanx region. These two pulleys are essential for achieving good movements after reconstruction. Hence, sparing these two pulley segments, the other segments may be opened up to allow access to the tunnel. Through the approaches possible, a hemostat should be passed gently to dilate the space in the tunnel that has collapsed and also to release some of the adhesions that are holding the walls together. By this method, most of the tunnel can be recreated. However, the proximal part may be difficult to clear, because it contains the densely adherent proximal edges of the tendons.
- Now, a longitudinal incision should be made on the forearm measuring about 5 to 6 cm, about 2 cm proximal to the wrist crease. This incision should be on the ulnar half of the distal forearm.
- The flexor digitorum superficialis (FDS) and FDP tendons of the fingers should be dissected through this incision. Care should be taken to avoid injury to the median nerve at this area.
- Take a polyethylene tube—a scalp vein set tube with the needle end cut-off. Thread the free end of the tube in to the carpal tunnel from the palm. Retrieve the tube in the proximal end in the forearm and retain it with a hemostat. Route this palmar end of the tube further distally through the remaining flexor tendon sheath to the insertion of the FDP tendon. The polyethylene tube now lies in the proximal course of the tendon implant
- Change the gloves, wash with normal saline and open the tendon implant packet.

> Make sure that glove powder does not come in contact with the implant material. If so, talc granuloma may form and cause adhesions.

- Now, attach the tendon implant to the proximal end of this polyethylene tube with 4.0 polypropylenes using horizontal mattress suture. Now, gently pull on the distal end of the polyethylene tube to railroad the tendon implant through the entire length, to the point of distal tendon edge at the terminal phalanx. Now, the entire tendon implant has been positioned (Fig. 4.14.2).

15 Flexor Tenolysis

Introduction

One of the most rewarding surgeries of the tendons is flexor tenolysis. This surgery is done when the passive range of motion is more than the active range of motion.

Presurgical Counseling

- This procedure will be done under wrist block anesthesia as patient cooperation will be required in the course of the procedure.
- A tourniquet will be applied and raised, but will be released before pain starts.
- This procedure will take about 30 to 45 minutes to perform if it involves a single finger and more if more fingers are involved.
- The return of full movement will be shown to the patient on the table. If this movement is to be maintained, postoperative physiotherapy is a must.
- A dressing will be applied and no plaster of Paris (POP) will be applied.
- A catheter will be placed in the wrist (like an IV cannula), through which, anesthetic solution will be injected if there is pain.
- Admission will be necessary for a minimum period of 3 days.
- Postoperatively, gentle active mobilization of the finger should be continued. If it is stopped, the finger will get back to the original state before surgery.
- In some instances, if the tendon is very grossly stuck and devoid of blood supply, a staged reconstruction may have to be done. This involves inserting a tendon implant, harvesting a tendon graft, and two surgical stages.
- In some instances, in the postoperative period, the tendon may rupture due to reduced blood supply. In such situations, the aforementioned staged procedure will have to be done after the wounds heal.
- In some instances, even if the movements of the finger improve, further surgery may be required to reconstruct the pulleys.
- The general complications of local anesthetic infiltration like hypersensitivity may occur in spite of test dose application. This complication will cause dryness of mouth and apprehension, which can be corrected immediately.

Surgical Steps

- This procedure should be done under wrist block anesthesia. However, if more than one finger is involved, the procedure is better done under axillary block anesthesia, as the patient cannot tolerate the tourniquet for a prolonged time under local anesthesia.
- First prepare the hand as described in Appendix I.
- *Marking the incisions (Fig. 4.15.1):*

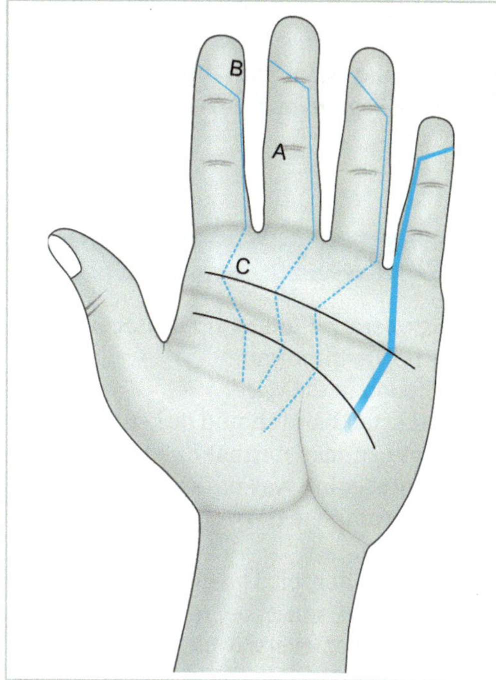

Fig. 4.15.1 Markings for exposure of the flexor tendons for tenolysis

- First make a marking 'A' on the neutral line of the noncontact surface of the finger from the web region to the distal interphalangeal (DIP) joint crease. This means that the incision should be made on the ulnar side for the index, middle and ring fingers and the radial side for the little finger.
- From the DIP joint crease level, extend the incision distally across the volar aspect of the terminal phalangeal segment (pulp region) in an oblique manner to reach the opposite side of the finger near the tip 'B'.
- From the point on the web region, extend the incision proximally 'C' in an oblique manner to reach the distal palmar crease. This marking will have to be extended proximally to reach the proximal part of the hollow between the thenar and hypothenar eminences.
- If multiple fingers are involved, multiple 'C' incisions cannot be made as the intervening skin flap may be jeopardized. Hence, a single 'C' incision to afford exposure of all the finger flaxors in the palm is advised.
- Make the incisions down to the subcutaneous tissue. On the neutral line segment and the terminal phalanx region, take care to avoid injuring the digital neurovascular bundle. Raise the entire skin and soft tissues of the volar aspect of the finger. Thus, the digital neurovascular bundle on the noncontact surface of the finger will be retained on the finger and the flap will be raised superficial to it. The flap continues to be raised superficial to the fibrous flexor sheath. This dissection stops when the digital neurovascular bundle of the opposite side of the finger comes into view.
- Now, raise the palmar portion of the flap along with the fat pad (superficial to the palmar aponeurosis). The noncontact side neurovascular bundle and the flexor tendon sheath will be visible on the bed.
- Anchor the raised skin flaps with 3.0 Ethilon after applying gentle traction on the skin flaps to afford maximal exposure of the entire flexor tendon sheath of the finger.
- All the adhesions between the tendons and the surrounding tissues must be divided. Care must be taken to avoid injuring the pulley system.
- When all the adhesions have been divided, the tendons must be pulled proximally and the movement of the finger noted. The finger must flex fully and the tip of the finger should touch the palm. If not, a few more adhesions will have to be released till this is achieved. Then ask the patient to flex the finger. He may not be able to isolate the finger to move due to the local anesthesia, so he must be instructed to flex all the fingers at once, slowly. This will flex the finger that is involved. The range of motion must be noted again. If all adhesions have been achieved, full range of active motion will be present. This must be shown to

the patient, so that it will serve as an impetus for postoperative physiotherapy. If full range is not achieved, two things are possible. Either there are more adhesions proximally, that should be released, or, the pulley system is damaged and needs to be reconstructed. This reconstruction should be done at a later procedure, since mobilization is needed after tenolysis, which cannot be implemented if pulley reconstruction is done.

- Moist saline gauze is placed over the entire length of the wound and gentle compression applied. The hand is elevated and the tourniquet released. After 3 minutes, the hand is kept back on the table and hemostasis achieved.
- For giving postoperative analgesia for the thumb, index and middle fingers, a Venflon catheter should be inserted in the volar aspect of the wrist, about 1 cm proximal to the wrist crease. The needle must be inserted to the ulnar side of the palmaris longus tendon, the needle being aimed deeply, pointing to the knuckle of the middle finger. This cannula will deliver anesthetic solution in the area surrounding the median nerve. If the ring or little fingers have been involved, the Venflon catheter is placed to the radial side of the flexor carpi ulnaris (FCU) tendon about 1 cm proximal to the wrist crease. This cannula must be fixed with plaster after the wounds are sutured.
- Suture the skin with 4.0 Ethilon after keeping Segmüller drains and apply sterile dressings.

Postoperative Protocol

The postoperative follow-up protocol of this surgery is very important.

- Admission in the ward.
- The affected hand should be kept elevated.
- Patient can take normal diet immediately if the procedure was under regional block or after complete recovery if under general anesthesia.
- Four milliliter of 1 percent solution of Bupivacaine must be injected into the cannula once every 6 hours. The patient must be attended to by a physiotherapist and both active and passive mobilization of the fingers must be done.
- Inspection of the suture line after 48 hours.
- Discharge of the patient by third day.
- Suture removal on the 10th day.
    - Refer to physiotherapy for active mobilization of the fingers
    - Daily wash with soap and water
    - Massage of scar and grafted skin with coconut oil.

Extensor Tendon Reconstruction

16

Introduction

In situations where there is a loss of extensor tendons on the dorsum of the hand, reconstruction with grafting is ideal since the extensor muscles are intact. If the extensor muscles are lost or deservated, tendon transfer is ideal and has been described in chapter 45.

Presurgical Counseling

- This procedure will be done under axillary block anesthesia or general anesthesia.
- The procedure consists of harvesting a tendon graft from either the forearm (in case of one or two fingers) and from the thigh (in case of more than two fingers).
- This procedure will take about 1½–2 hours to perform.
- A dressing will be applied and a plaster of Paris (POP) slab will be applied at the end of surgery.
- Admission will be necessary for a minimum period of 3 days.
- Postoperatively, no movements of the fingers should be attempted. If it is done, the sutured tendons may rupture.
- Postoperatively, the POP slab will be continued for a period of 3 weeks. After this period, physiotherapy will be started and this should be done for another 3 weeks.
- In some instances, even if the movements of the finger improve, further surgery may be required to release the scars that may form.
- The general complications of anesthetic infiltration like hypersensitivity may occur in spite of test dose application. This complication will cause dryness of mouth and apprehension, which can be corrected immediately.

Surgical Steps

- First the hand is prepared as described in Appendix I.
- *Markings for the incisions* will depend on the situation.
- There are two situations in which extensor tendon grafts are commonly done:
  - An injury to the extensor tendons on the dorsum of the hand with scars running across the dorsum of the hand or the forearm. These patients have presented late for treatment (more than 3 months). Hence, a secondary repair of the tendons will not be possible and a tendon grafting is done.
  - An injury with loss of extensor tendons on the dorsum of the hand with concomitant skin loss, which has been corrected by a skin flap surgery done at the time of injury. In such situations, the tendon reconstruction is done as a secondary procedure.
- In the former situation (Fig. 4.16.1), the incision is a longitudinally oriented lazy "S" shaped incision extending from about 4 cm distal to the scar to 4 cm proximal to the scar. The original scar is usually not

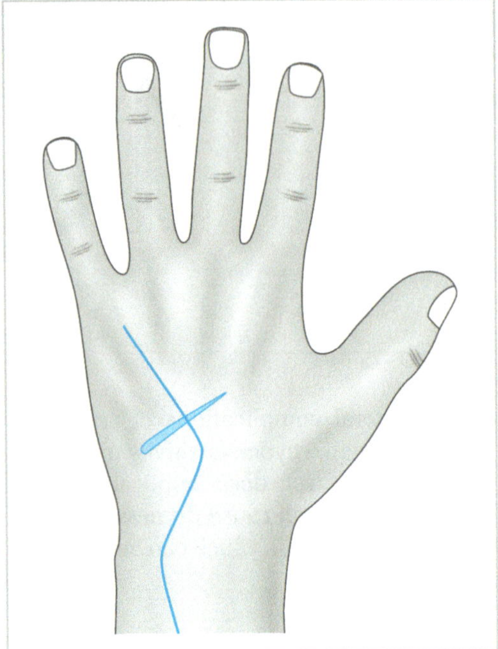

Fig. 4.16.1 Incision for extensor reconstruction

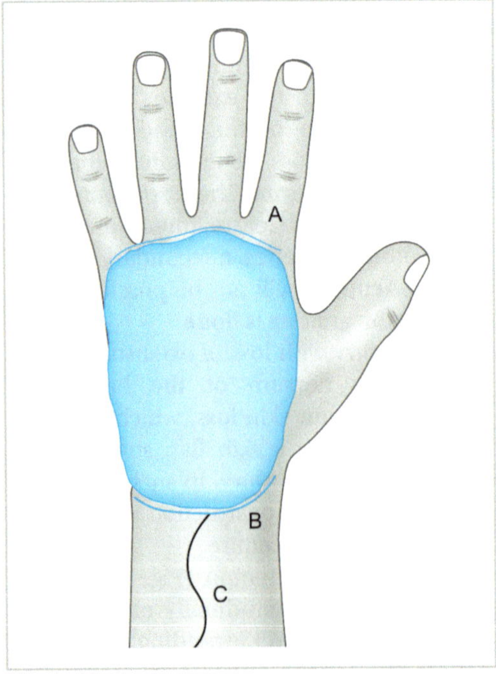

Fig. 4.16.2 Incisions in case of flap reconstruction

opened up and the new incision usually cuts across the previous scar.

- In the latter situation, where there is a skin flap over the area of tendon loss, the incisions are made as follows (Fig. 4.16.2):
  - The distal edge of the flap is marked "A" from the lateral side to the medial side.
  - The proximal edge of the flap is also marked "B" from the lateral side to the medial side.
  - From the center point of the proximal edge, an "S" shaped incision is marked "C", extending proximally for about 4 cm.
- The tourniquet is raised and the incisions are made as depends on the nature of injury as described above.
- First the distal incision is made. The skin flaps are dissected to afford good exposure of the distal ends of the extensor tendons. These tendons are isolated and all the scar tissues around them are excised. The tendons are pulled proximally with hemostats to determine whether the full range of passive movement has been achieved. If the finger movement is not full, further tenolysis must be done and the scars that attach the tendons to the bed must be released.
- Now, the proximal incision is made and the skin flaps reflected as marked. The proximal cut end of the extensor tendons are identified and dissected. The scars adherent to the proximal cut end of the tendons is excised. The tendons should be totally freed from scars and then the tendons should be pulled distally to evaluate the mobility of the extensor muscles. If the muscles are good, the tendon grafting can be done.
- The distance between the proximal end of the extensor tendons and the distal end is measured and the tendon graft harvested. If the tendon graft is planned for one or two fingers, the palmaris longus can be harvested as a graft. If the tendon graft is planned for more than two fingers, the palmaris longus may not be sufficient, and the fascia lata must be harvested as a graft.
- The method of harvesting the tendon grafts is described in Appendix VII and VIII.

- Tendon anastomoses using the palmaris longus tendon graft: the proximal tendon anastomosis is done first. The tendon graft is woven into the proximal cut ends of the extensor tendons with 4.0 polypropylene suture using horizontal mattress suture. After the tendon graft is woven through the ends of the tendons, the tendon graft is sutured to itself to make the anastomosis secure. Now, the distal end of the tendon graft is taken to the distal incision site. If the tendon graft is intended for two fingers, the tendon graft is split longitudinally. If this surgery is being done on a patient who has had a skin flap applied on the dorsum of the hand, the entire skin bridge need not be opened up. A subcutaneous tunnel can be created under the skin flap from the proximal incision to the distal incision. The tendon graft can be routed through this tunnel to the distal incision.
- If the fascia lata has been harvested as a tendon graft, the graft must be prepared before the proximal tendon anastomosis. The graft should be tubed with the external surface of the fascia lata graft going inside and the deeper surface of the graft forming the surface of the tube. The tubing is done after the formed tube is placed around the proximal ends of the cut extensor tendons. The seam line of the tube is sutured with 4.0 polypropylene using continuous buried suture technique. The tubing is not done for the entire length of the graft. The distal half of the tendon graft is split into slips depending on the number of fingers for which the extensors are to be reconstructed. The distal ends of the tendon graft are taken to the distal incision.
- *Distal tendon anastomoses:* The slips of the tendon graft are sutured to the distal ends of extensor tendons. The suturing is done with 4.0 polypropylene using horizontal mattress suture. At this juncture, the most important thing to consider is adjusting the tension of suturing. Each finger extensor must be sutured and the position of the finger checked. The tenodesis effect must be present. This means that when the wrist is flexed passively, the finger whose extensor has been repaired must extend passively. Similarly, when the wrist is extended, the finger must extend at the metacarpophalangeal (MCP) joint. Thus, the extensor tendons must be anastomosed for all the fingers after checking this effect.
- After all the extensors have been anastomosed, moist gauze is placed over the incisions, gentle compression applied and the hand elevated. The tourniquet is released, and the elevation of the hand is maintained for 3 minutes.
- The hand is then placed back on the table and hemostasis achieved. The wounds are sutured with 4.0 Ethilon after keeping Segmüller drains. Sterile dressings are applied.
- A volar slab POP is applied keeping the wrist in 30° extensions, the MCP joints in 60° flexion and the interphalangeal (IP) joints extended.

Postoperative Protocol

- Admission in the ward
- The affected hand should be kept elevated
- Patient can take normal diet immediately if the procedure was under regional block or after complete recovery if under general anesthesia
- Inspection of the suture line after 48 hours without disturbing the position of the POP slab
- Discharge of the patient by third day
- Suture removal on the 10th day
- Patient to retain the POP slab
- Removal of the POP slab on the 21st day and advise the following:
  - Refer to physiotherapy for active mobilization of the fingers
  - Daily wash with soap and water
  - Massage of scar and grafted skin with coconut oil
  - Patient is advised to continue the mobilization of the fingers; both active and passive and review once every month for evaluation.

Extensor Indicis Proprius to Extensor Pollicis Longus Tendon Transfer

17

Introduction

As described earlier, the loss of a segment of EPL tendon or delayed presentation of EPL tendon injury warrants reconstruction with a tendon transfer using EIP tendon.

Presurgical Counseling

- This procedure will be done under axillary block anesthesia or general anesthesia.
- The procedure consists of harvesting a tendon graft from the index finger. There will be no deficit on the index finger as a result of this.
- This procedure will take about 1½–2 hours to perform.
- A dressing will be applied and a plaster of Paris (POP) slab will be applied at the end of surgery.
- Admission will be necessary for a minimum period of 3 days.
- Postoperatively, no movements of the fingers should be attempted. If it is done, the sutured tendons may rupture.
- Postoperatively, the POP slab will be continued for a period of 3 weeks. After this period, physiotherapy will be started and this should be done for another 3 weeks.
- In some instances, even if the movements of the finger improve, further surgery may be required to release the scars that may form.
- The general complications of anesthetic infiltration like hypersensitivity may occur in spite of test dose application. This complication will cause dryness of mouth and apprehension, which can be corrected immediately.

Surgical Steps

- First the hand is prepared as described in Appendix I.
- *Markings for the incisions (Fig. 4.17.1):*

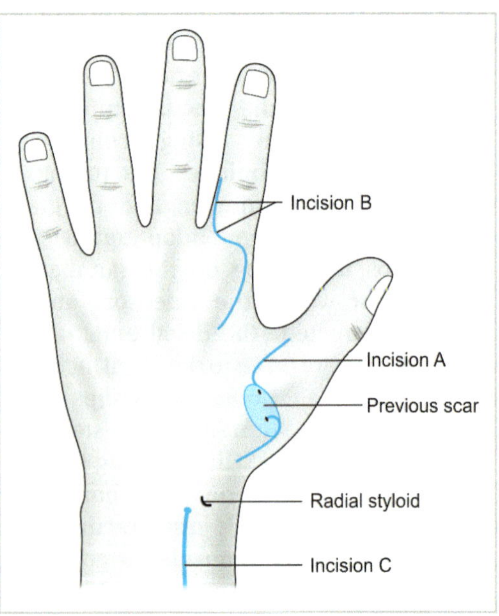

Fig. 4.17.1 Markings for the tendon transfer

- *Incision A:* An incision is marked over the area where the distal cut end of the extensor pollicis longus (EPL) tendon is present
- *Incision B:* Now, an S-shaped incision is marked over the dorsum of the proximal phalanx of the index finger, starting on the ulnar side of the proximal phalanx, extending proximally across the knuckle of the metacarpophalangeal (MCP) joint and the dorsum of the hand
- *Incision C:* Another incision about 2 cm is marked over the dorsal aspect of the wrist.

- The tourniquet is raised. First the incision to expose the EPL is made and the skin flaps are raised. The distal cut end of the EPL tendon is identified, and dissected free from the surrounding scar tissue. The EPL tendon is now pulled proximally after grasping with a hemostat. The passive movement of the thumb interphalangeal (IP) joint must be full. If it is not so, a further dissection must be done to release the tendon from the scar. The distance from the radial styloid to the dorsum of the IP joint of the thumb is measured. This will be the length of the extensor indicis proprius (EIP) tendon required beyond the wrist.
- Now, the incision is made to harvest the EIP tendon. The skin flaps are raised and anchored with 4.0 Ethilon sutures. The extensor tendons to the index finger are exposed. Now, the EIP tendon is isolated. Of the two extensor tendons to the index finger, the ulnar side tendon is the EIP tendon. The tendons are separate from each other till they reach the knuckle of the index. An incision is made over the middle of the extensor expansion, and extended distally for as much length of the tendon is required.
- Now, the tendon of EIP is harvested. It is pulled distally to confirm that there are no more attachments of the EIP. Now, the incision "C" is made and the EIP tendon pulled out through this wound.
- Now, a subcutaneous tunnel is created between the incision "A" and incision "C". A tendon retriever is inserted from the incision "A" and passed through the subcutaneous tunnel to the incision "C". Here, the free end of the EIP tendon is grasped, pulled and delivered at incision "A".
- Moist gauze is placed over the wounds and gentle compression is applied. The hand is raised and the tourniquet released. The elevation of the hand is maintained for 3 minutes and then the hand is placed back on the table. Hemostasis is achieved.
- The gap that has been created in the extensor apparatus by the removal of the EIP tendon is sutured with 4.0 polypropylenes using continuous suture. The skin wounds at incision "B" are sutured with 4.0 Ethilon.
- The skin wounds at incision "C" are also sutured with 4.0 Ethilon after securing hemostasis.
- Now, the distal end of the EIP tendon must be sutured to the EPL tendon. The mechanical advantage is more if the EIP tendon is sutured as distally as possible. If a long length of the EPL tendon is available, it is advantageous to excise a portion of this tendon up to the level of the MCP joint of the thumb and then suture the EIP tendon to the remaining stump of the EPL tendon. A trial stitch with 4.0 polypropylenes is applied and the tension is checked. The tenodesis effect is now checked as an indicator of the tension adjustment in the tendon anastomosis. The wrist is passively flexed. This movement should cause extension of the thumb IP joint. Similarly, passive flexion of the wrist should cause a flexion of the thumb joints. If this happens, the tension on the tendon transfer is correct. If there is too much tension, or too little tension, it should be corrected by redoing the tendon anastomosis.
  - The tendon anastomosis is done by Pulvertaft weave. Hold the EPL tendon taut with a hemostat applied on the end and pulling proximally.

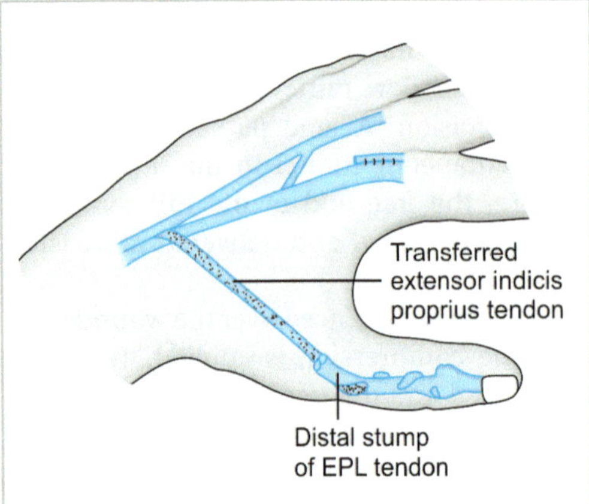

Fig. 4.17.2 Completed tendon transfer

- About 1 cm proximal to the end of the tendon, make a cut in a volar to dorsal direction with a number 11 blade, with just enough length to allow the tendon graft through. Pull the tendon graft through and adjust the tension so that the finger lies in the normal cascade. Apply a suture with 3.0 polypropylene using horizontal mattress suture (Fig. 4.17.2).
- About 1 cm proximal to the first cut, make another cut with number 11 blade, from a radial to ulnar direction. Thread the free end of the tendon graft through this opening also and suture with 3.0 polypropylenes using horizontal mattress suture.

- When the tendon anastomosis is over, the extra length of the EIP and EPL are trimmed. Wound closed with 4.0 Ethilon sutures.
- Moist saline gauze is placed over the entire length of the wound and gentle compression applied. The hand is elevated and the tourniquet released. After 3 minutes, the hand is kept back on the table and hemostasis achieved.
- Sterile dressings are applied and a volar POP slab should be applied for the hand keeping the wrist in 30° extension, and the MCP joints of the fingers in flexion of 90° and IP joints in extension and a POP slab for the thumb keeping the IP joints in extension.

Postoperative Protocol

- Admission in the ward
- The affected hand should be kept elevated
- Patient can take normal diet immediately if the procedure was under regional block or after complete recovery if under general anesthesia
- Inspection of the suture line after 48 hours without disturbing the position of the POP slab
- Discharge of the patient by third day
- Suture removal on the 10th day
- Patient to retain the POP slab
- *Removal of the POP slab on the 21st day and advise the following:*
    - Refer to physiotherapy for active mobilization of the fingers
    - Daily wash with soap and water
    - Massage of scar and grafted skin with coconut oil
    - Patient is advised to continue the mobilization of the fingers; both active and passive and review once every month for evaluation.

> During the physiotherapy regime, concentrate first on getting back full range of active movements at the index finger (donor finger)!

Flexor Digitorum Superficialis to Flexor Pollicis Longus Tendon Transfer

18

Introduction

The loss of a segment of FPL tendon or delayed presentation of FPL tendon injury are best managed with a tendon transfer of the FDS of ring finger.

Presurgical Counseling

- This procedure will be done under axillary block anesthesia or general anesthesia.
- The procedure consists of harvesting a tendon graft from the ring finger. There will be minimal deficit on the ring finger as a result of this.
- This procedure will take about 1½–2 hours to perform.
- A dressing will be applied and a plaster of Paris (POP) slab will be applied at the end of surgery.
- Admission will be necessary for a minimum period of 3 days.
- Postoperatively, no movements of the fingers should be attempted. If it is done, the sutured tendons may rupture.
- Postoperatively, the POP slab will be continued for a period of 3 weeks. After this period, physiotherapy will be started and this should be done for another 3 weeks.
- In some instances, even if the movements of the finger improve, further surgery may be required to release the scars that may form.
- The general complications of anesthetic infiltration like hypersensitivity may occur in spite of test dose application. This complication will cause dryness of mouth and apprehension, which can be corrected immediately.

Surgical Steps

- First the hand is prepared as described in Appendix I.
- *Markings for the incisions (Fig. 4.18.1):*
  - *Incision A:* A zig-zag incision is marked over the volar aspect of the proximal phalanx region of the thumb, where the flexor pollicis longus (FPL) tendon can be dissected

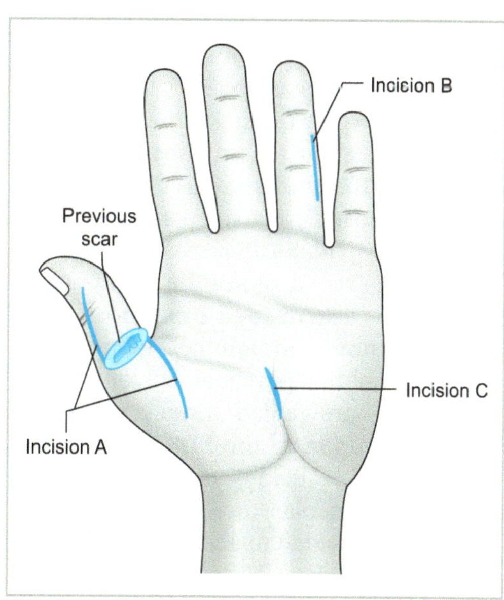

Fig. 4.18.1 Markings for the incisions

  - *Incision B:* Now, an incision is marked over the neutral line on the ulnar border of the ring finger about 4 cm long, centered at the level of the proximal interphalangeal (PIP) joint crease. This incision is to divide the insertion of the flexor digitorum superficialis (FDS) of the ring finger
  - *Incision C:* Another incision about 2 cm is marked over the palm in the proximal part of the hollow between the hypothenar and thenar eminences.
- The tourniquet is raised. First the incision to expose the FPL is made and the skin flaps are raised. The distal cut end of the FPL tendon is identified, and dissected free from the surrounding scar tissue. The FPL tendon is now pulled proximally after grasping with a hemostat. The passive movement of the thumb interphalangeal (IP) joint must be full. If it is not so, a further dissection must be done to release the tendon from the scar.
- Now, the incision "B" is made to harvest the FDS tendon. The skin on the volar side is raised superficial to the digital neurovascular bundle. The flexor tendon heath is identified. An incision is made in the flexor tendon sheath to isolate the FDP and FDS tendons. The FDP tendon is usually seen first and it must be retracted volarward to expose the FDS tendon slips. The ulnar slip is first seen. A hemostat is applied about 1 cm proximal to the insertion. The tendon slip is now cut distal to the hemostat. Now, traction is applied to this cut slip with the hemostat and this will expose the radial slip of the FDS tendon. This slip is also divided 1 cm proximal to the insertion and another hemostat is applied on the proximal cut end. Both hemostats are pulled distally to expose the decussation of the FDS tendon. It is divided with a blade until both slips are free. The vincular attachment will also have to be divided to achieve total release of the FDS slips.

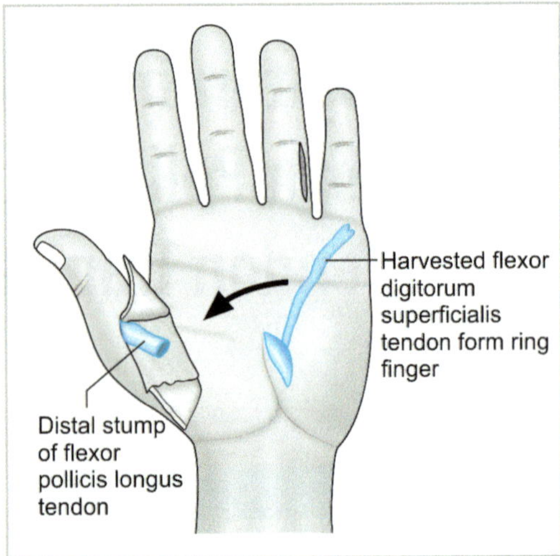

Fig. 4.18.2 Harvested FDS tendon ready for transfer

- Now, the tendon of FDS is ready for harvest. It is pulled distally to confirm that there are no more attachments of the FDS. Now, the incision "C" is made and the FDS tendon pulled out through this wound (Fig. 4.18.2).
- A subcutaneous tunnel is created between the incision "A" and incision "C". A tendon retriever is inserted from the incision "A" and passed through the subcutaneous tunnel to the incision "C". Here, the free end of the FDS tendon is grasped, pulled and delivered at incision "A".
- Moist gauze is placed over the wounds and gentle compression is applied. The hand is raised and the tourniquet released. The elevation of the hand is maintained for 3 minutes and then the hand is placed back on the table. Hemostasis is achieved.
- The skin wounds at incision "B" are sutured with 4.0 Ethilon.
- The skin wounds at incision "C" are also sutured with 4.0 Ethilon after securing hemostasis.
- Now, the distal end of the FDS tendon must be sutured to the FPL tendon. The mechanical advantage is more if the FDS tendon is sutured as distally as possible. If a long length of the FPL tendon is

available, it is advantageous to excise a portion of this tendon up to the level of the IP joint of the thumb and then suture the FDS tendon to the remaining stump of the FPL tendon. A trial stitch with 4.0 polypropylenes is applied and the tension is checked. The tenodesis effect is now checked as an indicator of the tension adjustment in the tendon anastomosis. The wrist is passively flexed. This movement should cause extension of the thumb IP joint. Similarly, passive flexion of the wrist should cause a flexion of the thumb joints. If this happens, the tension on the tendon transfer is correct. If there is too much tension, or too little tension, it should be corrected by redoing the tendon anastomosis. The tendon anastomosis is done by modified Kessler Mason suture using 3.0 polypropylene suture materials.

- When the tendon anastomosis is over, the extra length of the EIP and EPL are trimmed. Wound closed with 4.0 Ethilon sutures.
- Moist saline gauze is placed over the entire length of the wound and gentle compression applied. The hand is elevated and the tourniquet released. After 3 minutes, the hand is kept back on the table and hemostasis achieved.
- Sterile dressings are applied and a dorsal POP slab should be applied for the hand keeping the wrist in neutral, and the metacarpophalangeal (MCP) joints of the fingers in flexion of 90° and IP joints in extension and a dorsal POP slab for the thumb keeping the IP joints in 15° flexion and the MCP joint in 15° flexion and the carpometacarpal joint in palmar abduction.

Postoperative Protocol

- Admission in the ward
- The affected hand should be kept elevated
- Patient can take normal diet immediately if the procedure was under regional block or after complete recovery if under general anesthesia
- Inspection of the suture line after 48 hours without disturbing the position of the POP slab
- Discharge of the patient by third day
- Suture removal on the 10th day
- Patient to retain the POP slab
- Removal of the POP slab on the 21st day and advise the following:
    - Refer to physiotherapy for active mobilization of the fingers
    - Daily wash with soap and water
    - Massage of scar and grafted skin with coconut oil
    - Patient is advised to continue the mobilization of the fingers; both active and passive and review once every month for evaluation.

> The procedure done has transferred a powerful tendon to do a relatively light work.
>
> Hence, the movement of the thumb may be seen quite early into the physiotherapy!

SECTION 5

Bone Reconstruction

Bone Reconstruction—Assessment

19

Introduction

When there is an evidence of bone problem, the evaluation of the patient will be directed to find the nature of the problem and deciding on a plan of management. It must be remembered that a problem of the bone may result in alteration of the function of the other structures like the tendons and joints. Hence, an evaluation should assess not only the bone problem *per se,* but also the effects of the problem affecting the other structures in the hand.

History

Nature of Injury

The nature of injury will give a clue about the magnitude of the problem. A low-energy injury may cause a fracture but the effect may be negligible on the surrounding structures like tendons and joints.

Duration

If an injury has occurred more than 2 weeks earlier, the bone is probably beginning to unite and the callus has formed. If the fracture had been sustained less than 2 weeks back, it may need to support and immobilization.

Nature of Previous Management

This must be recorded. Any previous management, whether operative or otherwise, should be noted.

Skin

Presence of scars, protruding K-wires from previous treatment should also be noted.

Deformity

When there is a deformed part of the finger or hand, the cause is usually a malunited fracture. The points to be recorded are:

- *Site of the deformity:* It will point to the bone that has been injured
- *Angulation at the deformity:* This must be measured and recorded. Some fractures develop characteristic angulation due to the forces that act on the proximal and distal segments
- *Rotation at the deformity:* Some displaced fractures also get rotated and united in this deformed position. This deformity will be manifested by an altered orientation of the affected fingers with respect to the other fingers. This is recorded as an ulnar or radial rotation

Table 5.19.1 Planning the management schedule

Fracture	*Characteristic*	*Management*
Fracture of finger proximal phalanx (PPX) or middle phalanx (MPX) or metacarpal less than 2 weeks old	Good position	Immobilize in plaster of Paris (POP) slab
	Unacceptable position	Open reduction internal fixation (ORIF)
	With loss	Bone grafting
Fracture of finger PPX or MPX or metacarpal 2–4 weeks old	Good position	Mobilize the finger
	Unacceptable position	ORIF
	With loss	Bone grafting
Fracture of finger PPX or MPX or metacarpal greater than 4 weeks old	Good position	Mobilization
	Unacceptable position	Mobilize to make the proximal and distal joints supple Then take up for refracturing and fixation
	Loss involving segment of single bone	Bone graft from ulna
	Loss involving greater than one bone	Vascularized bone graft from fibula

- *Tenderness/signs of inflammation:* These may be present in addition to deformity when there is an evidence of infection in the involved bone
- *Range of motion (ROM) at the joints:* The problem of the bone can affect the joints and tendons of the affected finger or hand. These problems can be diagnosed by measuring and recording the active and passive range of movements at the various joints. When the active range of movement is less than the passive range of movements, it indicates that the tendons have become adherent to the fracture site. If the passive range of motion is restricted, it indicates that the joint itself may be involved by stiffness or ankylosis
- *Shortening of the hand/fingers:* The deformity of the bone, apart from producing angulation and rotation, can also produce shortening of the finger.

Sinus

- *Location of the sinus:* It will indicate the bone involved
- *Type of discharge:* A serous discharge may indicate an inflammatory reaction within the bone. A purulent discharge will indicate a frank infection
- *Surrounding skin:* Inflammatory changes/eczema may be seen in the surrounding skin.

Abnormal Mobility

- Site of abnormal mobility
- Tenderness.

Management

Planning the management schedule is given in Table 5.19.1:

Open Reduction Internal Fixation of Fractures

20

Introduction

Unacceptable position of union of fractures of the bones of hand require open reduction and fixation, such position leads to gross shortening of the finger/rotation leading to scissoring of the fingers while making a fist, or gross deformity. Such deformities lead to biomechanical disturbances that compromise function of the hand.

Presurgical Counseling

- This procedure will be done under axillary block anesthesia or under GA (in children).
- This procedure will take about 2 hours to perform.
- Wires will have to be introduced into the bone to fix it in the correct position.
- A dressing and a plaster of Paris (POP) will be applied.
- Admission will be necessary for a minimum period of 3 days.
- Postoperatively, no movements of the fingers should be attempted. The POP slab must be retained for a minimum period of 3 weeks. After the period of 3 weeks, the wires will be removed from the hand after confirming the healing with appropriate X-rays. Even before the wires are removed, physiotherapy may be required. After the wires are removed, it is necessary to undergo a period of physiotherapy till good movements are achieved.
- During the period of physiotherapy, splints may have to be applied as considered to appropriate by the surgeon/physiatrist.
- This surgical procedure aims only at getting the deformity/fracture corrected. Any injury of the surrounding structures will be dealt with later.
- In some instances, if the movements of the fingers do not return fully, a minor surgery may have to be done to release the stuck flexor or extensor tendons.
- The general complications of local anesthetic infiltration like hypersensitivity may occur in spite of test dose application. This complication will cause dryness of mouth and apprehension, which can be corrected immediately.

Surgical Steps

- Prepare the hand as described in Appendix I.
- Mark a cross finger flap like incision on the dorsum of the proximal phalanx (PPX) or middle phalanx (MPX) region of the finger (Fig. 5.20.1). If there is already a scar on the finger, it can be incorporated in to the incision. If a metacarpal bone is involved, the incision is made on the dorsum of the hand over the metacarpal.

the point of entry of the wire with local anesthetic solution. Now, advise the following:

- Refer to physiotherapy for active mobilization of the fingers
- Daily wash with soap and water
- Massage of scar and grafted skin with coconut oil
- Patient is advised to continue the mobilization of the fingers; both active and passive and review once every month for evaluation.

Vascularized Fibula Transfer

22

Introduction

Reconstructive surgery on the hand can never be completed without the vascularized fibula flap in surgeons armamentarium. The use of this technique is wide and the main indications are:

- Traumatic segmental loss
- Osteomyelitis
- Low grade malignant bone tumors
- Locally aggressive bone tumors
- Epiphyseal arrest due to trauma/infection.

Presurgical Counseling

- This procedure will be done under axillary block anesthesia and general or spinal anesthesia.
- This procedure will take about 6 hours to perform.
- This procedure will entail removing a piece of bone from the leg along with its blood supply and fixing it inside the hand to replace the bone. This will entail a vascular anastomosis procedure. There will be no deficit due to removal of the bone graft from the leg.
- A dressing and a plaster of Paris (POP) will be applied both on the hand and the leg.
- Admission will be necessary for a minimum period of 1 week.
- Postoperatively, no movements of the fingers should be attempted. The POP slab must be retained for a minimum period of 3 weeks. After the period of 3 weeks, the wires will be removed from the hand after confirming the healing with appropriate X-rays. After the wires are removed, it is necessary to undergo a period of physiotherapy till good movements are achieved.
- During the period of physiotherapy, splints may have to be applied as considered to appropriate by the surgeon/physiatrist.
- This surgical procedure aims only at getting the deformity/fracture corrected. Any injury of the surrounding structures will be dealt with later.
- In some instances, if the movements of the fingers do not return fully, a minor surgery may have to be done to release the stuck flexor or extensor tendons.
- The general complications of local anesthetic infiltration like hypersensitivity may occur in spite of test dose application. This complication will cause dryness of mouth and apprehension, which can be corrected immediately.

Surgical Steps

- The preferred anesthesia is either general anesthesia or combined regional block—continuous epidural anesthesia with supra-clavicular block (if the surgery is for finger or hand motorization).
- Prepare for the procedure as outlined in the Appendix II.
- Prepare the involved upper limb, including the shoulder, neck, front of chest.

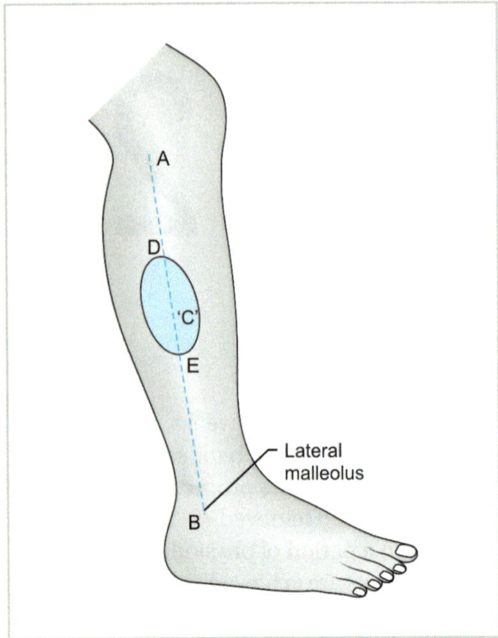

Fig. 5.22.1 Markings for raising the flap

- Prepare the opposite side thigh and leg and foot regions.
- *Markings for the flap (Fig. 5.22.1):*
  - Mark a point "A" on the fibular head. Mark a point "B" on the lateral malleolus. Join these two lines. This line AB forms the axis of the flap. It represents the underlying fibula position
  - Mark the midpoint "C" of the line AB. This point "C" represents approximately the area where the nutrient artery enters the fibula
  - Mark the skin paddle of the flap. This should be in the form of an ellipse, with the proximal and distal ends "D" and "E" lying on the axis AB. The maximum dimensions of the flap can be up to 15 cm × 8 cm.
- Positioning of the patient—flex the hip to about 60°, flex the knee to about 135°, and internally rotate the leg.
- First make the incision on the anterior border of the flap, from the points "D" to "E". This incision should go down to the deep fascia, incise it and stop when the peroneal muscles are seen. Now, elevate the flap from anterior to posterior over the peroneal muscles. As you do this, you may find a few musculocutaneous perforators from the muscle to the skin. These perforators can be ligated and divided. The elevation of the flap should stop at the posterior edge of the peroneal muscles or when the intermuscular septum is reached. This is the posterior intermuscular septum between the peroneal muscles and the soleus muscle, and it is this septum that contains the septocutaneous perforators to supply the skin paddle.
- Now, make the posterior incision. This incision should also go through the deep fascia and stop on the surface of the soleus muscle. Raise the skin paddle from the posterior to the anterior direction over the soleus muscle. A few perforators will be encountered, going from the muscle to the skin flap (Fig. 5.22.2).

  These perforators can also be ligated and divided. The dissection stops when the posterior surface of the posterior intermuscular septum is reached.
- Now, go back to the anterior surface of the intermuscular septum. Divide the

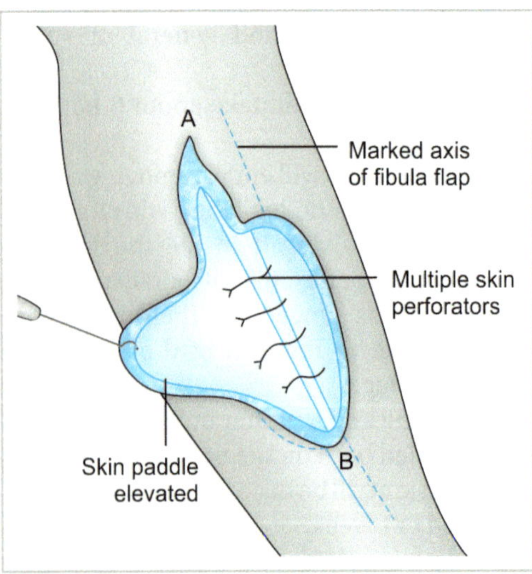

Fig. 5.22.2 Perforators entering the skin flap

peroneal muscles from the fibula bone along the entire length from "D" to "E". Do not divide too close to the bone, but leave a cuff of muscle on the bone. As this is being done, the dissection will go anteriorly on the anterolateral surface of the fibula. This dissection will stop at another intermuscular septum. This is the anterior intermuscular septum between the peroneal muscles and the extensor muscle compartment.

- This septum can also be divided and the extensor compartment will be reached. If the extensor muscles are retracted, the anterior tibial vascular bundle can be seen. Now, continue to dissect closing to the fibula. The interosseous membrane will now be opened and the tibialis posterior muscle encountered. When this muscle is retracted, the peroneal vascular bundle will be seen. The entire length of the peroneal vessels must be dissected. The branches from the artery to the fibula and the nutrient vessel can be seen. This dissection should be done in a plane deep to the peroneal vessels and not between the fibula and vascular bundle. The plane of the vessels is shown in Figure 5.22.3.
- The posterior dissection along the soleus muscle should be continued now. Keep dividing the soleus muscle fibers and freeing the muscle from the fibula and the intermuscular septum. Now, the entire length of the posterior intermuscular septum can be dissected. The proximal and distal osteotomies can be done now. Further dissection can be completed after the osteotomy.
- Mark the site of the proximal osteotomy. Make the incision in the periosteum about 2 cm proximal to this site. Elevate the periosteum up to the site of the proposed osteotomy. Carry out the osteotomy.
- Mark the site of distal osteotomy. Make an incision on the periosteum and then perform the osteotomy.
- Now, the osteotomized bone segment and the skin paddle will be attached by the posterior intermuscular septum, the peroneal vascular bundle and a few fibers of the flexor hallucis longus muscle. These fibers can be retained along with the pedicle to prevent injury to the vessels.

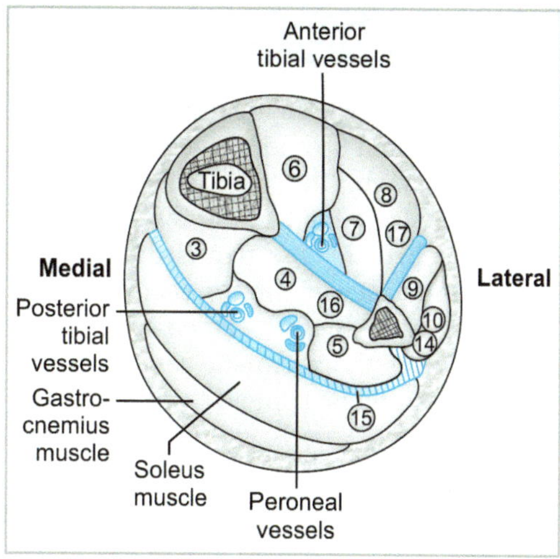

Fig. 5.22.3 Cross-section of leg showing the relative anatomy
Key: 3. Flexor digitorum longus; 4. Tibialis posterior; 5. Flexor hallucis longus; 6. Tibialis anterior; 7. Extensor hallucis longus; 8. Extensor digitorum longus; 9. Peroneus brevis; 10. Peroneus longus; 14. Fibula; 15. Transverse intermuscular septum; 16. Interosseous membrane; 17. Anterior intermuscular septum

- The fibular osteocutaneous flap is now ready for transfer. The division of pedicle should be done only after the completion of the dissection in the recipient site.
- *Division of the pedicle:* Usually, there are two veins and one artery at the vascular pedicle and the nerve. Soft clamps should be applied over the artery and veins. The proximal ends of the artery and veins should be ligated with 3.0 Vicryl. The vessels should be divided and the time noted. The flap should be placed on a moist abdominal pad and taken to the recipient site for vascular anastomosis.
- *Management of the donor site:* After securing hemostasis, the secondary defect should be closed with a skin graft from the thigh. Sterile dressings should be applied and elastocrépe bandage applied over it. A posterior below knee slab is applied.

Vascular Anastomosis

- The flap is brought to the hand defect. First the flap is held up and the pedicle allowed to hang down. This step will make sure that there is no inadvertent twisting of the vascular pedicle. The flap is then placed over the defect with the correct orientation and the end of the pedicle should be placed over the recipient vessels. A few sutures should be applied to inset the flap.
- The recipient vessels should be divided, blood flow checked from the divided artery and approximator clamps applied. The soft clamps must be released from the donor vessels. Vascular anastomosis should be done (the technique of vascular anastomosis is beyond the scope of this manual).

Postoperative Protocol

- Admission in the ward for a minimum period of 1 week
- The affected hand and the leg should be kept elevated
- Patient can take normal diet immediately if the procedure was under regional block or after complete recovery if under general anesthesia
- Inspection of the suture line after 48 hours without disturbing the position of the POP slab
- Suture removal on the 10th day
- Patient to retain the POP slab
- Removal of the POP slab from leg on the 21st day. Take an X-ray of the part to confirm the healing of the bone on hand. If the X-ray shows a good healing, the K-wire can be removed in the operation theater after infiltrating the point of entry of the wire with local anesthetic solution. Now, advise the following:
  - Refer to physiotherapy for active mobilization of the fingers
  - Daily wash with soap and water
  - Massage of scar and grafted skin with coconut oil
  - Patient is advised to continue the mobilization of the fingers; both active and passive and review once every month for evaluation.

SECTION

6

Joint Reconstruction

Joint Reconstruction—Assessment

23

Introduction

When a patient presents with a problem of the joint, assessment of the situation should lead to the cause of the problem. The assessment of a joint is twofold. The joint could either have been injured *per se* or it could have become involved after an injury which is not directly on the joint.

This section deals mainly with post-traumatic sequelae affecting the joints. Conditions like tumors, degenerative diseases like rheumatoid disease, and congenital anomalies can also affect the joints, but such problems are not highlighted in this chapter.

Clinical Examination

The examination of the patient should follow the steps outlined below:

- *Cause of the injury:*
    - Blunt injuries are likely to cause dislocations and closed fractures. It should be noted whether this type of injury has caused an injury to the joint. Even an injury at a remote site can result in a stiffness of the joint of the hand. This should also be recorded.
    - Open injuries are more likely to cause soft tissue disruption which may cause instability of the joint.
- *Duration of the injury:* This is very important. When a dislocation of the proximal interphalangeal (PIP) joint occurs, and the patient presents within a week to 10 days, the chances of achieving a good reduction and hence good function are high. However, if the patient presents later than this period, it is more likely that the function of the joint may have been lost forever.
- *Local symptoms:* Like pain or swelling can occur in situations where there is inflammation
    - Infection of the joint can occur after penetrating injuries like human bite.
    - Inflammation can occur following vigorous, unsupervised physiotherapy.
    - The management of both these conditions is different and hence the correct diagnosis is essential.
- *Constitutional symptoms:* Like fever and malaise may occur when there is a hematogenous spread of infection from a joint.
- *Position of the joint:* It is important to record the resting position of the joint as it gives a clue to the underlying pathology.
    - *Associated fracture:* As mentioned earlier, the fracture of the proximal phalanx can cause a stiffness of the PIP joint, even if the fracture has not been intra-articular. This is caused mainly by improper position of the joints during immobilization at the time of treatment of the fracture.
- The range of movements of the joint must be recorded. This will include both active and passive range of movement. This recording has two uses:

- Daily wash with soap and water.
- Massage of scar and grafted skin with coconut oil.
- Prescribe a dynamic knuckle bender splint to be worn 24 hours a day for a further 3 weeks.
- Review after this period. If the active range of movement is full, discard the splint. If the range of movement is not full, to continue wearing the splint at night for a further 3 weeks.

Vascularized Toe Metatarsophalangeal Joint Transfer

26

Introduction

When the joint of a finger has been destroyed, the resulting function in the finger is compromised. Replacement of the joint by biological, vascularized tissue is perhaps the ideal reconstruction in such cases. Disadvantages that are seen for artificial joint replacement are not seen in this method of microvascular reconstruction.

Presurgical Counseling

- This procedure will be done under axillary block anesthesia for the hand and general or spinal anesthesia.
- This procedure will take about 6 hours to perform.
- This procedure will entail removing a joint from the second toe of the leg on the same side as the hand injured, along with its blood supply and fixing it inside the injured finger to make the new joint heal properly. This will entail a vascular anastomosis procedure. After the joint is removed, the second toe will have to be shortened and the wound closed primarily. There will be no deficit in walking due to removal of the joint and loss of toe.
- A dressing and a plaster of Paris (POP) will be applied both on the hand and the leg.
- Admission will be necessary for a minimum period of 1 week.
- Postoperatively, no movements of the fingers should be attempted. The POP slab must be retained for a minimum period of 3 weeks. After the period of 3 weeks, the wires will be removed from the hand after confirming the healing with appropriate X-rays. After the wires are removed, it is necessary to undergo a period of physiotherapy till good movements are achieved.
- During the period of physiotherapy, splints may have to be applied as considered appropriate by the surgeon/physiatrist.
- This surgical procedure aims only at getting the deformity/fracture corrected. Any injury of the surrounding structures will be dealt with later.
- In some instances, if the movements of the fingers do not return fully, a minor surgery may have to be done to release the stuck flexor or extensor tendons.
- The general complications of local anesthetic infiltration like hypersensitivity may occur in spite of test dose application. This complication will cause dryness of mouth and apprehension, which can be corrected immediately.

Preparation

- Palpate the dorsalis pedis artery and mark the course.
- Put the leg in a dependent position and mark the main dorsal veins, the transverse arch and the great saphenous system.
- Mark a point "A" at the level of the distal edge of the inferior extensor retinaculum,

halfway between the dorsalis pedis artery marking and the great saphenous system marking.

- Draw a curvilinear line between the point "A" and the web space between the great toe and the second toe.
- Similarly, from the web space between the great toe and second toe, on the plantar aspect, make a marking that extends from the apex proximally along the second metatarsal to the midsole.
- If a skin flap is needed, it can be planned on the dorsum of the metatarsophalangeal (MTP) joint of the second toe. The flap should not extend distal to the level of the proximal interphalangeal (PIP) joint.

Surgical Steps

- Prepare for the surgery as described in the Appendix I and II.
- Make the dorsal incision down to the dermis only.
- Raise medial and lateral flaps for about 2 to 3 cm on either side.
- The following should be dissected now—the great saphenous vein, other dorsal veins, fat and subcutaneous tissue.
- Dissect the dorsalis pedis artery up to the distal part of the intermetatarsal space, where it will divide into two branches to the great toe and the second toe.
- Dissect the deep peroneal nerve and divide it at the level of the MTP joint of the second toe. It is not required in the flap.
- At the distal part of the first dorsal metacarpal artery, identify the deep communicating branch going to the plantar side. This branch will join with the first plantar metatarsal artery to form the plantar digital artery. And this plantar digital artery will divide into two, the medial plantar digital artery going to the lateral side of great toe and the lateral plantar digital artery going to the second toe. Examine this system to see which is dominant—the first dorsal metatarsal artery and the dorsal digital arteries or the first plantar metatarsal arteries and the plantar digital arteries.
- Now, surgeons go to the plantar side dissection. Make the plantar incisions. The plantar incision is needed only if the vessels cannot be clearly dissected from the dorsal approach.
- The medial plantar digital artery (branch to the great toe) is divided.
- The transverse metatarsal ligament is divided on the lateral aspect of the MTP joint of the second toe. This should be done as close to the joint as possible without injuring the capsule.
- Now, retractors should be applied to the second metatarsal and retracted laterally and the first metatarsal retracted medially. The arterial system is now exposed. The system should be carefully dissected, taking into account the dominance of the vessel system. This can be assisted by carefully dividing the interosseous muscles and further exposing the arterial system.
- Now, disarticulate the second toe at the level of the PIP joint. Now, the MTP joint of the second toe is almost completely dissected and is held only by the intact metatarsal bone and the artery and veins. The osteotomy of the metatarsal can be done. This should be done depending on the length that surgeons have already calculated in the preoperative work-up.
- The osteotomy should be done in an oblique manner. This is because of the nature of the MTP joint of the toe. This joint is basically an extension joint. The range of motion of this joint is 0–550 of extension and 0–50 of flexion. If this joint is used to replace any of the small joints of the hand, it will not be physiological, because the joints of the hand should have more amount of flexion and lesser amount of extension for good function. Hence, the MTP joint of the toe must be modified, if it is to become a flexion joint

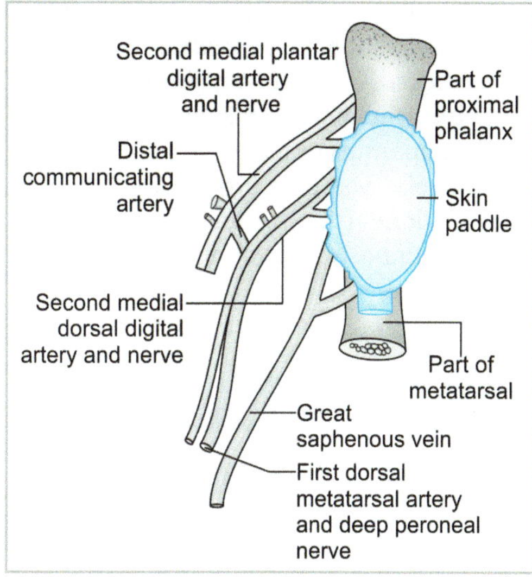

Fig. 6.26.1 Harvested second toe MTP joint, ready for transfer

in the hand. The easiest way to do this is to do an oblique osteotomy at the neck of the metatarsal bone.

- The next step is to make transverse drill holes on the metatarsal and the proximal phalanx adjoining the joint. Stainless steel wire (24G) are threaded through these drill holes and kept ready.
- Once the osteotomy is over, the remaining soft tissues can be divided, so that the second toe joint is now held only by the arteries and veins (Fig. 6.26.1).
- Now, release the tourniquet, apply warm, moist pads over the second toe and the vascular pedicle. Take care to prevent the toe from falling down and shearing the vessels! Raise the foot for about 5 minutes. Then place the foot on the table. It usually takes about 15 to 20 minutes for the circulation to be re-established in the dissected skin flap. By the end of this time, the flap becomes pink and warm and ready for transfer.

> It is very important to ensure the wait till the toe becomes pink and warm. It may take quite some time (half an hour even) before this happens. During this time, the surgeon can prepare the recipient site, or if it has already been done, can go for a coffee break and prayer!

- The vessels can be divided when the recipient site dissection is over.
- *Division of the pedicle:* Soft clamps should be applied over the artery and veins. The proximal ends of the artery and veins should be ligated with 3.0 Vicryl. The vessels should be divided and the time noted. The flap should be placed on a moist abdominal pad and taken to the recipient site for vascular anastomosis.
- *Management of the donor site:* After securing hemostasis, the second toe must be shortened and the wound closed primarily in layers with 3.0 Vicryl for the subcutaneous tissues and 4.0 Ethilon for skin. Drainage tubes should be placed. Sterile dressings should be applied and elastocrépe bandage applied over it. A posterior below knee POP slab should be applied.

Recipient Site Dissection

- The hand is prepared as described in Appendix I
- A curvilinear incision is made over the anatomical snuff box area and the following structures are identified and dissected:
  - The radial artery and both venae comitantes
  - The cephalic vein
- One percent of Xylocaine gauze is applied over the dissected vessels
- A volar incision is made on the stump of the thumb proximally up to the thenar area. Raise the medial and lateral skin flaps,

apply anchoring sutures with 3.0 Ethilon and dissect the following structures:
  - Prepare the ends of the bony stumps to which the MTP joint of the second toe is going to be fixed. Pass transverse drill holes through both ends of the bone which will lie proximal and distal to the position of the joint
- Apply gentle compression with moist gauze and padding over the wound. Release the tourniquet. Hold the hand in an elevated position for a period of 4 to 5 minutes. Rest the hand on the table and secure hemostasis.

Fixation of the Toe Metatarsophalangeal Joint Flap

- Bring the toe flap to the recipient site. Place the MTP joint of the toe in position, a position in which good function can be achieved with the fingers.
- A subcutaneous tunnel is created between the recipient site vessels and the summit of the stump. This tunnel is for the vessels of the toe to be passed through to reach the recipient vessels—the radial artery.
- The structures to be passed through the tunnel are:
  - The arteries
  - The veins
  - Bone fixation—fix the bones, both proximally and distally with the stainless steel wires that had already been passed. This can be done by using square knot of the wire without causing damage to the vessels.
  - Tendon repair—this may be required, in conditions of trauma only. In congenital conditions, the tendons will be intact and tendon reconstruction may not be necessary.
  - Vascular anastomosis—the recipient vessels should be divided, blood flow checked from the divided artery and approximator clamps applied. The soft clamps must be released from the donor vessels. Vascular anastomosis should be done (the technique of vascular anastomosis is beyond the scope of this manual).

Postoperative Protocol

- Admission in the ward for a minimum period of 1 week.
- The affected hand and the leg should be kept elevated.
- Patient can take normal diet immediately if the procedure was under regional block or after complete recovery if under general anesthesia.
- Inspection of the suture line after 48 hours without disturbing the position of the POP slab.
- Suture removal on the 10th day. Patient to retain the POP slab.
- Removal of the POP slab on the 21st day. Take an X-ray of the part to confirm the healing of the bone. If the X-ray shows a good healing, the K-wire can be removed in the operation theater after infiltrating the point of entry of the wire with local anesthetic solution. Now, advise the following:
  - Refer to physiotherapy for active mobilization of the fingers.
  - Daily wash with soap and water.
  - Massage of scar and grafted skin with coconut oil.
  - Patient is advised to continue the mobilization of the fingers; both active and passive and review once every month for evaluation.

SECTION

7

Nerve Reconstruction

Nerve Reconstruction—Assessment

27

When the patient has an injury to the nerves, the diagnosis may sometimes be quite obvious. When assessing such an injury, the effects of injury to the nerve can be seen in the hand, where, the neural deficit will be seen. This includes motor, sensory and autonomic neural deficits that must be assessed. The assessment of the deficits has been outlined in the chapter on Hansen's disease—assessment.

The injuries to the median, ulnar and radial nerves will be considered, and the methods of reconstruction will be dealt with. The functional deficit associated with each nerve is different. When the ulnar nerve is involved, the deficit is mainly in the power of the hand, and when the involvement is of the median nerve, it is more of a precision and fine work deficit that is noted. So, when a manual labourer presents with an ulnar nerve involvement, he is more likely to be incapacitated by the problem, than a person who is a sedentary worker with the same nerve involvement.

The next assessment should be of the specific motor or sensory deficit, because the treatment protocol will be aimed at correcting the particular problem. In a case of ulnar nerve injury, who has had a previous surgery, or has had a partial involvement only, there may be a sparing of some of the innervated muscles. In such a situation, it is not prudent to carry out the routinely described tendon transfers blindly.

All hands are not alike. We are likely to come across some patients with thin and fragile hands, and sometimes some patients with short stubby and thick hands. So it is obvious that any described tendon transfer will not have the same results in all types of hands. Hence, the assessment of the habitus of the hand must also be made, before planning the treatment protocol.

Nerve Reconstruction—Management

28

Approaches and Exploration

Points to be remembered when exploration is planned for nerve injury:

- It is not advisable to approach the deeper tissues through the scar that is present. This is because, the tissues will be grossly adherence at this area and it may be very difficult to identify the injured nerve in this scar tissue. The chances of inadvertent injury to the nerve are also possible.
- Hence, the incision should incorporate the scar in the standard prescribed incision for exploration of the particular nerve.
- The dissection of the nerve should commence in the area distal to the zone of injury and in the area proximal to the zone of injury, so that, the healthy nerve can be identified first and can then be traced to the area of injury.
- A liberal incision always helps in the following ways:
    - Tissue handling is more gentle and rough retraction is not required.
    - The exposure offered is better and gives an idea about the relative anatomy in the zone of exploration.
    - Thus, both time and energy are saved in this technique.

The markings for nerve exploration depend on the site of injury of the nerve. However, there are some standard incisions that are used when the nerves are explored.

In the arm:

- Radial nerve is approached by a longitudinal incision on the lateral aspect of the entire arm, over the palpable border of the humerus.
- Median nerve and ulnar nerve are approached by a longitudinal incision on the medial side of the entire length of the arm.

In the forearm:

- Median nerve and the ulnar nerve are approached by a lazy "S" incision on the flexor aspect of the forearm, from the elbow to the wrist crease.

In the palm:

- *Median nerve and ulnar nerve:* The incision should be made on the thenar crease.
- *Digital nerves in the palm:* Zig zag incisions on the palm.
- *Digital nerves in the fingers:* Neutral line incision on the appropriate side to expose the digital nerves.

Nerve Repair

- The hand is prepared as described in Appendix I
- The markings are made as described above.
- The tourniquet is raised and the skin incisions are made as planned.
- The incision is made down through the skin and subcutaneous tissues to the deep fascia of the forearm. This fascia is incised and the compartment of the flexor muscles

is reached. The muscles are dissected carefully and the median nerve is looked for in the plane between the flexor digitorum superficialis (FDS) and the flexor digitorum profundus (FDP). If there is any difficulty in locating the median nerve, it can be traced in a retrograde manner from the distal part of the forearm, where it is relatively easily identified among the tendons. The nerve lies deep to the palmaris longus tendon and to the radial side of the FDS and FDP tendons to the fingers. In the distal part of the forearm, opening the deep fascia will give access to the tendons.

- When the nerve has been dissected, the ends of the nerve are examined under microscope. There is usually a rounded swelling of the proximal end of the nerve which consists of the neuroma. There is a swelling on the distal end of the nerve constituting a glioma. Both these swellings must be excised before reconstruction of the nerve can be done.
- The excision of the neuroma should be done under the microscope. A scalpel handle is taken and totally wound with moist gauze piece over a length of about 5 cm. This part of the handle is then placed under the end of the nerve and the excision of the neuroma begins. With a number 11 blade, the neuroma is cut transversely across. The proximal end of the cut neuroma is examined under microscope, to look for evidence of fascicles. The fascicles will appear clearly only in the intact portion of the nerve. In other areas, the nerve fascicles will appear hazy and surrounded by homogenous scar tissue. The proximal end of the nerve should again be cut at a distance of 1 mm from the end. This end should again be examined for determining the integrity of the fascicles as described above. This process should be continuously done until anatomically intact fascicles are encountered. There should be absolutely no scar tissue in the end of the nerve now. On examining the epineurial covering of the nerve, blood vessels should be seen running on the surface till the cut end of the nerve. The nerve should feel soft and supple to the palpating finger. Now, the proximal end of the nerve is ready for reconstruction.
- This procedure should be repeated for the distal end also. By this, the distal end of the nerve will also be ready for reconstruction.
- Now, the process of mobilization of the nerve ends should be done. This is done to free the proximal and distal nerve segments from any scars that have formed with the surrounding soft tissues. This is done gently teasing the tissues around the proximal and distal nerve segments and freeing the nerves. It should be remembered that this process of mobilization should not be extended for more than 5 to 8 cm from both ends, as this may lead to devascularization of the nerve segments.
- The nerve ends should be placed loosely on their bed and the reconstruction plan should be made:
    - Ends of the nerves are close to each other or gap less than 2 cm: primary repair of the nerve.
    - Gap between nerve ends between 2 and 10 cm: free nerve graft.
    - Gap between nerves ends greater than 10 cm: vascularized nerve graft.
- Primary repair of the nerve—the nerve ends are placed closing to each other and a background material is placed under the proposed site of nerve repair (this background material is available commercially). The ends of the nerve should fall in contact with each other when left lax. Hemostasis is achieved and then the orientation of the nerve ends is matched.
- The orientation of the fascicles is matched on the proximal and distal ends of the nerve.
- If blood vessels are seen running on the epineurial surface, these are matched between the proximal and distal ends.
- Now, the epineurial repair (Fig. 7.28.1) is done after orienting the cut ends correctly. The repair is done under microscope. In no

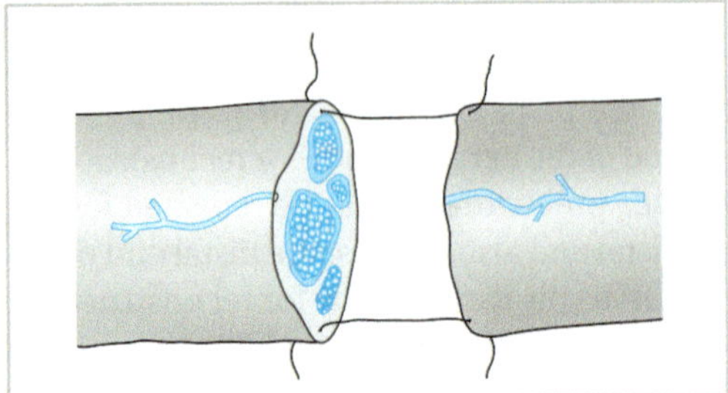

Fig. 7.28.1 Epineurial repair

part of the surgery should the nerve tissue be held with the forceps. The microsurgery instruments set is opened now and only these instruments are used. The suturing is done between the epineurium of the proximal end and the epineurium of the distal end with 8.0 Ethilon using simple interrupted sutures. This suturing is done around the circumference of the nerve.

Nerve Grafting

- The gap between the nerve ends is measured. The surface area of the cut ends of the nerve is assessed. Usually, about 3 cables of nerve graft will be required for the reconstruction of median nerve in the forearm and 2 cables for the ulnar nerve in the forearm. Hence, the requirement of nerve graft should be assessed carefully before harvesting the graft. The sural nerve is commonly harvested as a nerve graft and the procedure is described in Appendix IV.
- *Nerve graft anastomosis:* The first step done is to reverse the nerve graft. This is easily done by the following steps:
  - The nerve graft has a stitch of 7.0 polypropylene on the distal end (the end from the calf region of the leg). The other end of the graft is the proximal end.
  - Place the proximal end of the nerve graft at the cut end of the distal segment of the nerve. Place the entire length of the graft on the nerve gap and the bed. Suture the nerve graft to the distal cut end of the nerve as described above.
  - Now, cut the nerve graft at the point where it reaches the proximal end of the nerve and let this cut end of the graft stay near the proximal end of the nerve. Bring the remaining nerve graft again to the cut end of the distal segment of the nerve. Align them and suture by applying epineurial sutures as described above.
  - Cut the remaining nerve graft at the level of the proximal cut end of the nerve. Bring the remaining nerve graft to the cut distal end and repeat the process described above.
  - At the end of this step, the distal end of the nerve would have been sutured to three cables of the nerve graft, and the free ends of the three cables will be lying near the proximal cut end of the nerve. The free end of the third cable will still be showing the stay suture of 7.0 polypropylene.
  - Now, these three cables should be sutured to the proximal cut end of the nerve with 8.0 Ethilon epineurial sutures, starting with the deepest cable.
- The skin wound is now closed with 4.0 Ethilon after keeping Segmüller drainage tubes.
- Sterile dressings are applied and a plaster of Paris (POP) slab is applied, keeping the wrist in neutral position, and metacarpophalangeal (MCP) joints of fingers in flexion, the interphalangeal (IP) joints straight.

Postoperative Protocol

- Admission in the ward.
- The affected hand should be kept elevated.
- Patient can take normal diet immediately if the procedure was under regional block or after complete recovery if under general anesthesia.

- Analgesics and antibiotics for 5 days.
- Sedation sos for 1 day.
- Inspection of the dressing after 48 hours.
- Discharge of the patient by third day.
- Suture removal on the 10th day.
- Removal of the POP slab on the 14th day and advise the following:
- Refer to physiotherapy for active and passive mobilization of the fingers and thumb.
- Daily wash with soap and water.
- Massage of scar and grafted skin with coconut oil.
- Compression garment for scar softening after a further 2 weeks.

SECTION

8

Complex Post-traumatic Problems

Complex Post-traumatic Problems—Assessment

29

Introduction

The assessment and management of different structures of the hand have been discussed in the earlier segments. However, in practice, it is not always a problem of only the tendon, or only the joint and so on. It is usually a combination of problems that is present in a single hand. There may be an adherent scar on the dorsum of the hand and there may be a loss of extensor tendons on the fingers, along with malunited fractures of multiple metacarpal bones.

When such a patient presents, it may be difficult to go through each single chapter and then come to a diagnosis and form a plan of management. This chapter tries to consolidate the findings in the previous chapters in a single chart, to simplify evaluation.

In such situations, there are important goals to be achieved.

- The exact problem, i.e. the tissue problem must be assessed
- The nature of the problem must be assessed, i.e. whether there is a loss of tissue
- The management protocol must be decided
- The sequence of management must also be charted.

Skin:
- Presence of raw areas
- Presence of chronic ulcers/trophic ulcers
- Presence of scars
- Presence of grafted skin
- Presence of flaps
- Presence of contractures.

Tendon:
- Flexor/extensor
- Injury/segmental loss
- How many fingers are involved?

Nerve:
- Which nerve/nerves?
- What is the level of injury?
- What is the deficit?

Bone:
- Which bone?
- Which finger?
- *Nature of problem:* Malunion/nonunion.

Joint:
- Which joint/joints?
- Which finger/fingers?
- *Nature of problem:* Stiffness/ankylosis/instability.

Priority of Management

First Make a Plan According to Diagnosis

- *Skin:* First the plan for the skin reconstruction can be made according to the discussion in the Chapter 10
- *Tendon:* The plan is made according to the assessment done as described in Chapter 11
- *Nerve:* The plan is made as described in Chapter 27

- *Bone:* The plan is made as described in Chapter 19
- *Joint:* The plan is made as described in Chapter 23.

Now, the different plans have been made for the individual problems, they have to be integrated into a total solution and the timing has to be decided.

Classify According to Postoperative Regimen

- *Procedures that require immobilization:* Some procedures require immobilization after surgery, like reconstruction with nerve grafts, bone fixation, tendon grafts and tendon transfers, etc.
- *Procedures that require mobilization:* Some procedures require that mobilization be started immediately after the surgical procedure. Examples are procedures like arthrolysis and tenolysis.

Classify According to Time Schedule

- *Procedures that can be done immediately:* Some procedures have to be done immediately, like resurfacing of raw areas. These procedures should be planned as soon as possible after the required investigations are done and the raw area is fitted for surgical resurfacing
- *Procedures that have to be done later:* Some procedures like reconstruction of the tendons and nerves can be done as elective procedures after investigations are done and after the patient is adequately counseled about the various reconstructive options
- *Procedures that have to be done after the environment becomes conducive in the hand:* There are some procedures for which the timing can be planned only when the tissues are conducive. For example, tendon reconstruction cannot be done unless the joints of the hand and fingers are made adequately supple, either by physiotherapy or surgical maneuvers.

Classify According to Priority Lists

- If both upper limbs are involved, can both upper limbs be operated on together? If not, which hand to be operated first
- If multiple fingers are involved, can all fingers be operated together? If not, which finger to be operated on first
- When multiple tissues are involved, which tissue reconstruction gets priority?

Priority Lists

If Both Upper Limbs are Involved

The priority is to be decided depending on the nature of involvement, age of the patient, disability in the patient.

- *According to the nature of involvement:*
  - The upper limb with raw areas, ulcers get priority
  - Then comes nerve involvement; the limb with nerve involvement should be treated first.
- *According to the age of the patient:*
  - In adults, both upper limbs are not usually operated on together, because then, the patient becomes dependent and may cause inconvenience
  - In children, both hands can be operated on together.
- *According to the disability in the patient:*
  - If one upper limb is so involved that it does not participate in the activities of daily living, this limb must be operated on first
  - If both limbs are equally involved, it is better to operate on the nondominant side first, so that the patient can get used to the routine of surgery and the postoperative protocols. Patient will thus be better prepared when the dominant hand is operated upon
  - If both upper limbs have been involved so badly that both are not used for activities of daily living, the dominant hand should be operated on first.

If Multiple Fingers are Involved

The priority is to be decided based on the fingers involved, the nature of the involvement and the nature of surgical management required.

- *According to the finger involved:* If the fingers and the thumb are involved, it is ideal to reconstruct the fingers first and then plan the reconstruction on the thumb.
- *According to nature of involvement:*
    - The finger with raw areas, ulcers gets priority
    - Then comes nerve involvement; the limb with nerve involvement should be treated first
    - When there is a contracture, adherent scar on one finger, this finger gets priority and gets operated on before the other fingers are operated on.
- *According to the surgical management required:*
    - When one finger requires a surgical procedure which need immediate mobilization in the postoperative period, this finger is operated on first. The fingers that need immobilization in the postoperative period are dealt with at a later stage.
    - When all fingers require surgical procedures needing immobilization in the postoperative period, the finger requiring a bone surgery is operated on first (deformity correction first).

If Multiple Tissues are Involved (Table 8.29.1)

- The first priority is the skin problem; whether it is a raw area or contracture or adherent scar. This should be corrected first before the other structures are dealt with.
- Then, this should be the correction of deformity and the achievement of stability. Hence, the bony reconstruction must be planned next.
- Once stability is achieved, surgeons should now achieve full passive mobility. So, the next priority is getting the full range of movements in the joints with arthrolysis.

Table 8.29.1	Involvement of different tissues		
Tissue involved	***Problem***	***Plan***	***Points to remember***
Skin	Raw area	Resurfacing with skin graft/flap	As soon as possible
	Adherent scar	Excision and flap cover	Elective
	Contracture	Release and split skin grafting (SSG)/flap cover	Elective
	Cosmetic deformity only	Correction	Elective
Bone	Malunion	Refixation of fracture	First priority after skin raw areas management
	Nonunion	Bone grafting	First priority after skin raw areas management
Joint	Stiff joint	Arthrolysis	Needs postoperative mobilization
	Ankylosed joint	Arthrodesis	To give stability
Nerve	Injury	Exploration and nerve reconstruction	To be done before tendon reconstruction
Tendon	Loss	Tendon reconstruction	
	Adhesions	Tenolysis	Needs postoperative mobilization

- The next on the list is achievement of active mobility. However, getting active movements in anesthetic hand is very dangerous as it may lead to the development of trophic ulcers. Hence, the reconstruction of the nerves must be done prior to the reconstruction of the tendons.
- If both the extensor and flexor tendons need reconstruction, the extensor tendon reconstruction is planned to be done first and the flexor tendon reconstruction is done at a later stage.
- In reconstructing the hand to achieve active movements, the reconstruction of the extrinsic tendons must be achieved before the reconstruction of intrinsic motors with tendon transfers.

SECTION

9

Thumb Reconstruction

Principles and Decision Making in Thumb Reconstruction

30

Principles

Loss of a thumb is a debilitating condition that results in loss of function and hence earning capacity, especially for a manual laborer. Considering the fact that loss of thumb amounts to 40 percent disability; there are various procedures to reconstruct the thumb. However, a hand surgeon must consider various factors before deciding on a particular method.

Characters that an ideal thumb must have:

1. Length
2. Stability
3. Mobility
4. Sensation
5. Cosmesis
6. Free from pain.

These characteristics are discussed in the following:

1. *Length:* The optimum length for a functioning thumb when all the fingers are intact is up to the neck of the proximal phalanx. This will ensure that there is functional contact between the tips of the fingers and the reconstructed thumb. If the length is less than that, function will be compromised and useful function will not result. So, when planning for reconstruction of a thumb, it should be planned for a length up to the neck of the proximal phalanx of the intact thumb. When planning for a thumb in a hand where all the fingers are missing or short, a thumb equal in length to that of a normal thumb should be planned.
2. *Stability:* The reconstructed thumb should be stable and able to maintain its position in status quo. The position of the thumb must be physiological and not in the way of the moving fingers. This depends on the stability provided by the bones that make up the reconstructed thumb. Obviously, when a thumb is being reconstructed, it will have to comprise an underlying foundation of bones, which may be as free grafts or vascularized graft. For the reconstructed thumb to be stable, the bones that make up the thumb must be:
   - Stably fixed to the underlying stump
   - Fixed in a correct position for function.

   This is more relevant when there is a total loss of thumb, without a carpometacarpal joint. In such a situation, when a toe transfer is done, the position of fixation is very important at the radius or stump of the carpus.
3. *Mobility:* The normal thumb has three joints: (1) Carpometacarpal (CMC) joint (2) Metacarpophalangeal (MCP) joint and (3) Interphalangeal (IP) joint of the thumb. So, mobility of the thumb is normally dependent on the movement at these three joints. Among these joints, the most important is the CMC joint of the thumb. If surgeons plan to reconstruct a thumb, it would be ideal to have the movements at all three joints and hence

ideal to reconstruct all three joints. Since, it may be difficult to reconstruct all three joints, the order of priority is to have a functioning and mobile CMC joint, or if that is not possible, a functioning and mobile MCP joint.

4. *Sensation:* For a thumb to function normally, the grips of the hand involving the thumb should be intact. This means that the reconstructed thumb should be capable of taking part in two types of activities: (1) power grips and (2) precision grips. When precision grips are involved, it is important that the pulp of the thumb be sensate. Only then, grip strength can be assessed by the thumb. The other reason is that, the thumb, being involved in most of the movements of the hand, if the tip is insensate, it will be prone for trophic ulceration. So, when a thumb is reconstructed, it is imperative that sensation is provided for at least the pulp region and the tip to achieve the goal of providing a functioning thumb.
5. *Cosmesis:* The thumb occupies a very large space in the cortex of the brain. The thumb, being an important part of the hand is always in the vision field of the patient and that of the observer. Hence, it is important that the reconstructed thumb look like a thumb with all the components, like quality of dorsal skin, quality of pulp skin and nail complex. Although a meticulously reconstructed thumb can bring back function to the patient's hand, the patient may not be totally satisfied if it does not look cosmetically acceptable. If this happens, the patient may slowly stop using the reconstructed thumb as he may be ashamed of it, and gradually, even a moving thumb may become useless to the patient just because it is cosmetically not accepted.
6. *Freedom from pain:* If a thumb were to be reconstructed that is totally stable and without any movement, there would be no pain at all. On the other hand, such a thumb would be useless to the patient. Only if there is movement, there will be function. And if there is movement, there are bound to be reconstructed moving joints and ligaments which will be prone for strain and wear and tear, leading to pain and ultimately, disuse. Hence, reconstruction of a thumb must not provide mobility at the cost of pain. This will totally defeat surgeons' purpose of providing a useful and functioning thumb.

Decision Making

There are certain set protocols in deciding about what method to use for thumb reconstruction in a particular case. However, there are many factors to consider, before deciding the method of reconstruction for a patient.

General Factors

1. *Sex:* The method of reconstruction differs for males and females in certain aspects. The requirements for the male thumb are the capability for manual labor and lifting heavy weights, especially in a country like India, where the manual laborers are usually the victims of industrial accidents who lose their thumb. Hence, a stable post is required, with minimal movements, to allow for the power grips. However, for males who are pursuing white collar jobs, or those who work as typists or musicians, or females, the requirement is the reconstruction of a fairly mobile thumb, which should provide the precision grips like pulp-to-pulp pinch, tip-to-tip pinch, etc.
2. *Age:* The requirement in children is almost the same as adults with a few differences:
   - When the reconstruction is done early in life, the reconstructed thumb gets incorporated in the body image faster
   - The reconstructed thumb must have a potential for growth in children. A good example is the use of vascularized wrap around great toe flap in amputation at

the level of the MCP joint. In adults, it provides an excellent reconstruction method and cosmesis. Even in children, it provides good results, but the biggest disadvantage in the use of this flap in children is its lack of growth potential. Hence, a flap that can grow along with the child is chosen, like a vascularized second toe transfer.

3. *Occupation:* As mentioned earlier, manual laborers require a more stable reconstruction with the ability for power grips, whereas sedentary laborers require more mobile reconstruction. An example would be the choice of vascularized wraps around great toe flap in amputation at the level of the MCP joint for manual laborers. This may not be an ideal method of reconstruction for sedentary workers, due to the lack of IP and MCP joint movements. Thus, more movements can be provided by the choice of vascularized trimmed toe transfer that can provide both mobility and cosmesis.
4. *Socioeconomic status:* A developing nation like India, financial constraints pose a problem when deciding on the choice of thumb reconstruction. When there has been an amputation at the level of the MCP joint, and carpometacarpal joint mobility has been preserved, the choice rests between osteoplastic reconstruction and vascularized wrap around great toe flap. Both the procedures provide a functioning thumb. The former procedure may prove financially viable for a patient who is more worried about the cost factor than the cosmetic factor. Thus, the option of classical staged method must also be offered to the patient before a decision can be arrived at.
5. *Other medical illnesses:* For mentally unstable patients and elderly individuals, classical methods of reconstruction may not be ideal. Single staged procedures like free flaps are preferred in such situations.

Local Factors

1. *Hand dominance:* A similar type amputation on both the thumbs of a patient may warrant different methods of reconstruction on the dominant hand and nondominant hand. This may be a controversial topic, but it is generally more practical to decide for a more elaborate reconstruction on the dominant hand.
2. *Other fingers:* When all the fingers are absent or shortened, the method of reconstruction may be totally different. Other ancillary procedures like thumb web deepening may have to be combined with the prescribed methods of reconstruction to create a useful thumb.
3. *Condition of the rest of the upper limb:* This is applicable in a situation like the congenital condition of radial club hand. The thumb may be hypoplastic and may require reconstruction. The preferred method of reconstruction will be the procedure of pollicization. However, the procedure should not be done if there is no movement at the elbow, which is sometimes the associated symptom in such a condition. This is because a moving thumb cannot produce function if it cannot move to the rest of the body where it has to act.
4. *Remaining stump of thumb:* The prescribed method of reconstruction depends also on the level of amputation of the thumb. For purposes of simplicity, surgeons can divide the thumb into levels as follows:

Type I

Amputation at tip of the thumb to the proximal third of the nail complex:

- Requisites of reconstruction: Sensate tip
- *Preferred methods:*
    - For Transverse amputation: Lateral advancement flaps of Kütler
    - For volar oblique amputation: Innervated cross finger flap

- For dorsal oblique amputation: Volar advancement flap of Atasoy–Kleinert
- *For radial/ulnar oblique amputation Type I:* Oblique triangular flap
- *For radial/ulnar oblique amputation Type II:* Dorsal transposition flap

Type II

Amputation proximal to the proximal third of the nail complex to the neck of the proximal phalanx:

- Requisites of reconstruction:
  - Preservation of length
  - Sensate tip
  - Cosmesis
- Preferred methods:
  - Transverse amputations: Staged Island flap of Professor R Venkataswamy.
  - Amputations with more dorsal loss: First dorsal metacarpal artery flap
  - Amputations with more volar loss: Littler's neurovascular Island flap

Type III

Amputation proximal to the neck of the proximal phalanx, up to the MCP joint:

- Requisites of reconstruction:
  - Provide length
  - Stability
  - Sensate tip
  - Cosmesis.
- Preferred methods:
  - Osteoplastic reconstruction
  - Vascularized wrap around great toe transfer

Table 9.30.1 Levels of amputation, characteristic and their surgical options

Level of amputation	*Characteristic*	*Surgical option*
Amputation at tip of the thumb to the proximal third of the nail complex	Transverse amputation	Lateral advancement flaps of Kütler
	Volar oblique amputation	Lateral advancement flaps of Kütler
	Dorsal oblique amputation	Volar advancement flap of Atasoy–Kleinert
	Radial/ulnar oblique amputation Type I	Oblique triangular flap of Professor R Venkataswami
	Radial/ulnar oblique amputation Type II	Dorsal transposition flap
Amputation proximal to the proximal third of the nail complex to the neck of the proximal phalanx	Transverse amputations	Staged Island flap of Professor R Venkataswami
	Amputations with more dorsal loss	First dorsal metacarpal artery flap
	Amputations with more volar loss	Littler's neurovascular Island flap
Amputation proximal to the neck of the proximal phalanx, up to the metacarpophalangeal (MCP) joint	Patient not willing for toe transfer Expertise not available for microsurgery	Osteoplastic reconstruction
	Patient willing for microsurgery	Vascularized wrap around great toe transfer
	In children	Vascularized second toe transfer
Amputation proximal to the MCP joint to the base of the metacarpal bone with intact carpometacarpal joint	Expertise not available for microsurgery	Pollicization + opponensplasty
	Microsurgical expertise available	Vascularized second toe transfer + opponensplasty
Amputation through the carpometacarpal joint with destroyed joint	Expertise not available for microsurgery	Pollicization
	Microsurgical expertise available	Vascularized transmetatarsal second toe transfer

- Vascularized second toe transfer (in children)
- On-top plasty
- Distraction lengthening.

Type IV

Amputation proximal to the MCP joint to the base of the metacarpal bone with intact carpometacarpal joint:

- Requisites of reconstruction:
  - Provide length
  - Mobility
  - Stability
  - Sensate tip
  - Cosmesis.
- Preferred methods:
  - Vascularized transmetatarsal second toe transfer
  - Pollicization.
  - Any of the above + Tendon transfer for opponensplasty.

Type V

Amputation through the carpometacarpal joint with destroyed joint:

- Requisites of reconstruction:
  - Provide length
  - Mobility
  - Stability
  - Sensate tip
  - Cosmesis.
- Preferred methods:
  - Pollicization
  - Vascularized transmetatarsal second toe transfer.

Ancillary procedures like phalangization and deepening of thumb web are discussed under the management of mutilated hand.

Levels of amputation, characteristic and their surgical options have been discussed in details in Table 9.30.1.

- The above criteria will be filled by the use of the volar advancement flap, originally described by Atasoy.

Surgical Steps

1. Axillary block anesthesia is given. A tourniquet is applied on the arm.
2. The hand is painted and draped. The tourniquet is raised. The wound is debrided and defect measurement is taken (Figs 9.31.2A and B).
3. The defect will be in the form of a circle or transverse oval, with the amputated end of the bone protruding in the center of the defect. Mark the two edges of the nail stump as "A^1" and "B^1".
4. Now, on the free edge of the defect on the volar skin, mark two points "A" and "B" corresponding to the points "A^1" and "B^1". Mark a point "C" in the midvolar aspect of the IP joint crease of the thumb. The 3 points "A", "B" and "C" are joined together to form a triangle, the base being formed by the volar edge of the defect, the apex being pointed proximally.
5. The two sides of the flap are incised with a number 15 blade down to the dermis only, and the incision completed by turning around the apex at the DIP joint.
6. Now, the incision is gently deepened till the fat globules protrude through the incision site. A skin hook is applied on the leading edge of the flap, i.e. the edge of the defect and mild traction applied. While maintaining traction, the knife is used to gently incise the fibrous septae one by one. As this is being done, the flap can be felt and seen to advance slowly.
7. When the flap covers the defect, and the advancing edge AB reaches the point "A" and "B", mobilization of the flap should be stopped (Figs 9.31.3A and B).
8. The tourniquet should be released, viability of the flaps confirmed, and hemostasis achieved.
9. The leading edge of the flap should be sutured to the nail bed on the dorsal aspect, using 4.0 polyamide sutures. The sides of the flap should be sutured using 4.0 polyamides in a "Y" fashion. The longitudinal

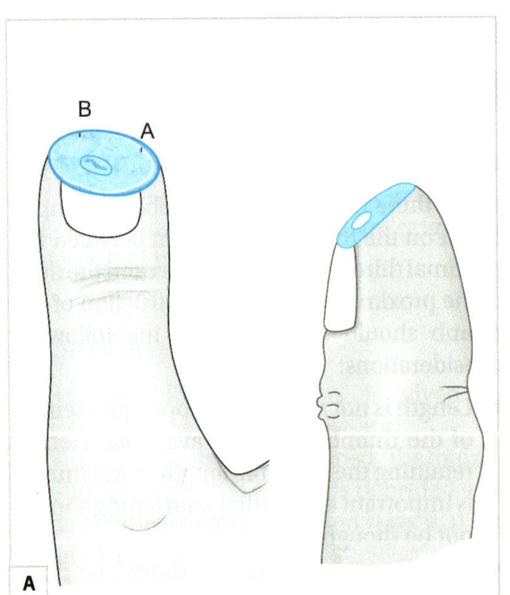

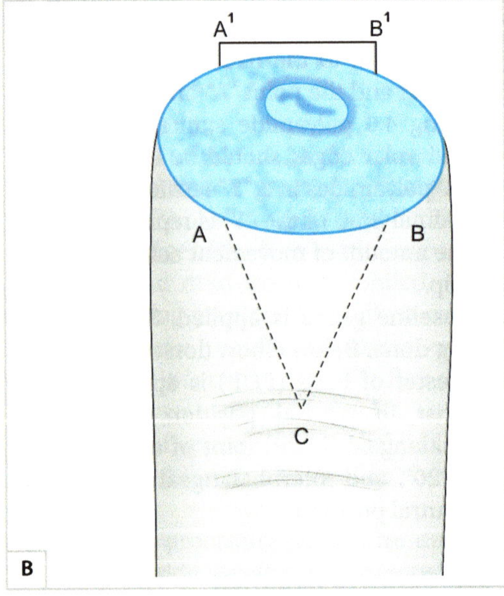

Figs 9.31.2A and B Defect and the markings for the flap

limb of the "Y" is representative of the amount of movement achieved by the flap.

10. Vaseline gauze is applied. Sterile dressing done. Below elbow dorsal slab thumb POP is applied with wrist in neutral position, MCP joint of thumb flexed at 20º, and IP joint in neutral position.

Postoperative Regimen

- *Day 2:* Inspection of flap and suture line
- *Day 10:* Suture removal, removal of POP slab, scar massage and mobilization of thumb.

Oblique Amputation Type "A"

Oblique Triangular Flap of Professor R Venkataswami

Oblique amputations on the thumb at Type I can be of two types. The classification depends on the angle of the obliquity. An oblique amputation means that there is more loss of one side, either the radial side or the ulnar side. Thus, one edge, either the radial or ulnar edge is more proximal. When the proximal edge of the amputation does not cross the level of the nail fold, the obliquity is minimal and is called oblique amputation type "A".

Surgical Steps

1. Axillary block anesthesia is given. A tourniquet to be tied on the arm.
2. Hand to be painted and draped. Tourniquet to be raised.
3. Debridement of the wound is done. The marking of the flap are now made. The points on the neutral line of the defect are marked. It will be seen that one point is more proximal than the other due to the obliquity of the defect. Mark this proximal point as "A". The distal point is marked "B". Now, a point "C" is marked on neutral line at the PIP joint on the side of point "B". These two points are joined by a line. Similarly "A" and "C" are joined. This line will cut across the IP joint crease. This is

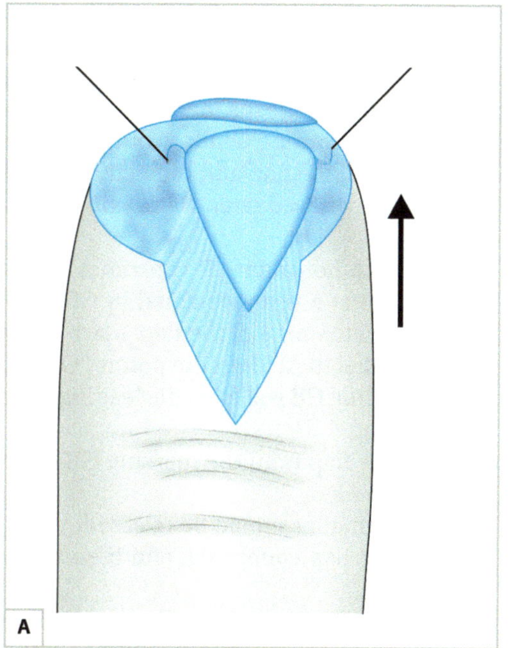

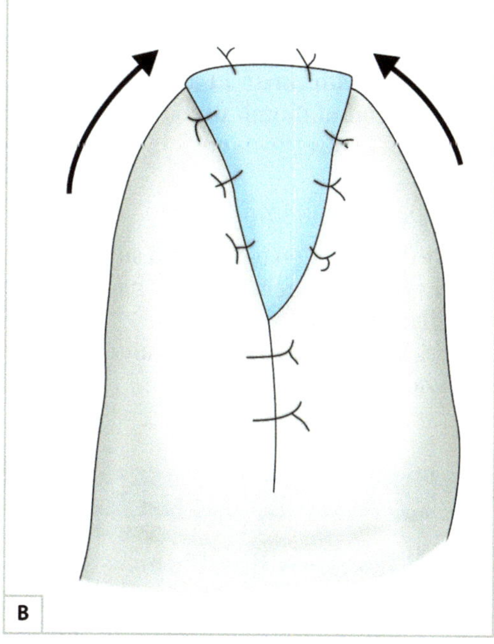

Figs 9.31.3A and B Showing the advancement of the flap and final suture line

marked as an oblique triangle with base on the edge of defect.

4. Make skin incision along BC and AC with number 15 blade. The incision is turned around the apex and completed.
5. Skin hooks are placed on the edge of the defect, and the flap is raised superficial to the fibrous flexor sheath. By doing this, the neurovascular bundle goes along with the flap. As it nears the apex, care should be taken not to injure the neurovascular bundle. When the flap is totally raised, it will be seen to be attached only by the neurovascular bundle. Now, the skin hooks are used to give gentle traction on the flap to advance it and the reach of the flap is checked.
6. Now, release the tourniquet, and secure hemostasis. Then inset the flap at the leading edge by using 4-0 polypropylene. Then the sides are sutured. It will be seen that the suture line is in the form of a "Y", the vertical limb of the "Y" denoting the amount of advancement of the flap.
7. Dressings are applied with vaseline gauze, dry gauze and finger dressings. Pad and bandage are applied on the hand and forearm.
8. Below elbow dorsal slab thumb POP is applied with wrist in neutral position, MCP joint of thumb flexed at 20°, and IP joint in neutral position.

Postoperative Regimen

- *Day 2:* Inspection of flap, and suture line
- *Day 10:* Suture removal is done, POP slab is discarded.

Advise: Wash with soap and water, massage scar and mobilize the thumb.

Oblique Amputation Type "B"

Dorsal Transposition Flap

As described, an oblique amputation may be of two types and will now discuss the optimal management of the second type. This type involves an obliquity in such a way that one end extends beyond the nail fold. Thus, the obliquity in this type of amputation is more than the obliquity in the first type.

Use of the dorsal skin as a transposition flap can be done by the following method.

Surgical Steps

1. Axillary block anesthesia is given. A tourniquet is applied on the arm.
2. The hand is painted and draped. The tourniquet is raised. The wound is debrided and defect measurement is taken (Figs 9.31.4A and B).
3. One edge of the oblique oval will be proximal to the nail fold, either on the radial side or on the ulnar side. Mark this point as "A". Mark the opposite end of the oval defect as "B". Measure the distance from "A" to "B". Measure the volar-dorsal distance at the widest point of the defect. Mark these points as "C" and "D" on the volar and dorsal sides respectively.
4. Mark this distance transversely on the dorsum of the terminal phalanx region, about 3 mm proximal to the nail fold, to protect the underlying hyponychium. This line may be at the point "A" or it may be 1 to 2 mm proximal to "A". This does not matter. It only means that there will be an intact skin bridge about 2 mm between the base of the flap and the defect, which has to be excised later. Name this line as AE.
5. Mark another point "F" proximal to the point "A" at a distance equal to CD. This will form the base of the flap. Mark a line FG parallel to AE. Join the points "G" and "E". The line GE will form the leading edge of the flap.
6. Raise the flap from the marking GE up to the base AF.
7. The tourniquet should be released, viability of the flap confirmed, and hemostasis achieved.
8. The leading edge of the flaps should be sutured to the distal edge of the defect and the sides of the flap should be sutured

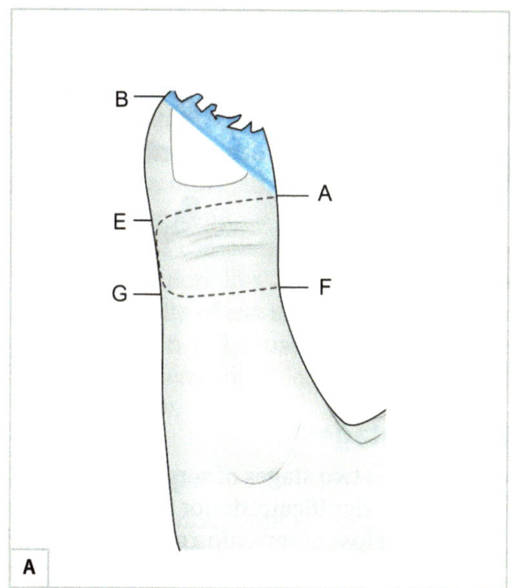

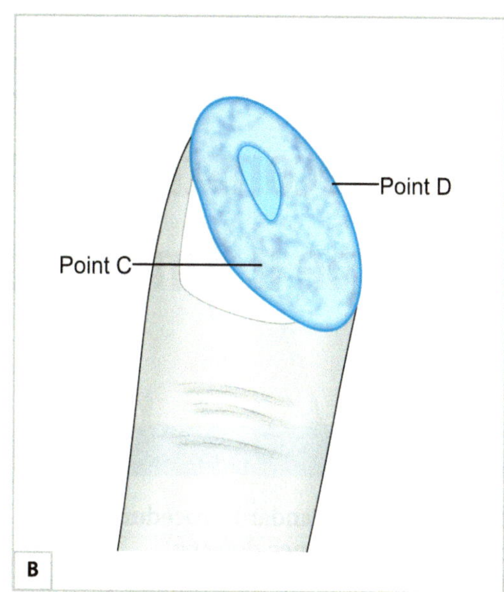

Figs 9.31.4A and B Markings for the dorsal transposition flap

to the volar and dorsal edges of the defect using 4.0 polyamide sutures.

9. *Management of the donor area:* After confirming hemostasis, the raw area on the dorsum should be covered with a split thickness skin graft. Now, raise the hand and prepare the arm with betadine solution. The skin graft should be harvested from the medial side of the arm. Sterile dressings should be applied over the skin graft donor site before moving back to the hand. The graft should be applied over the raw area and tie over sutures applied with 3.0 Ethilon.
10. Vaseline gauze is applied. Sterile dressing done. Below elbow dorsal slab thumb POP is applied with wrist in neutral position, MCP joint of thumb flexed at 20°, and IP joint in neutral position.

Postoperative Regimen

- *Day 2:* Inspection of flap and suture line
- *Day 10:* Suture removal, removal of POP slab, scar massage and mobilization of fingers.

dorsal side down to the extensor paratenon and the dorsal portion of the flap raised. Now, the distal margin of the flap incised and the neurovascular bundle ligated with 3.0 Vicryl and cut. The flap is now attached by the Grayson's and Cleland's ligaments. To divide these, the flap must be lifted up, the neurovascular bundle confirmed to enter the flap and the ligaments must be divided closing to the bone. This will free the flap some more.

8. As the base of the flap is reached, care should be exercised, as the neurovascular bundle is deep to this area. Gently free the neurovascular bundle from the deeper fibrous attachments and the multiple small branches coursing into the web. Now, the flap is free, attached only at the base "AB".
9. Gently move the flap to the defect over the skin to check whether it reaches the defect comfortably. If it does not, a little more dissection of the base of the flap is in order.
10. Apply wet gauze on the bed of the flap, xylocaine soaked gauze on the pedicle of the flap. Raise up the hand and release the tourniquet. Maintain the hand in elevated position for about 3 minutes and ask for the tourniquet to be removed entirely.
11. Now, set the hand on the table and examine the edges of the flap. There should be a slow and sustained subdermal bleed. This may not be evident immediately. It may take a few minutes for the spasm of the vessel to be relieved. In the meantime, continue to bathe the pedicle with 1 percent xylocaine solution and achieve hemostasis on the bed of the flap and the primary defect.

If there is no bleeding from the flap edges, look for any ligature of a branch that is too close to the vessel.

12. When good bleeding is seen from the edges of the flap, it is ready for insetting. Bring the thumb to the middle finger, so that the raw area is closed to the base of the flap "AB". Allow the flap to lie freely over the defect. When it does so, there is a raw area on the undersurface of the flap. It is not necessary to tube this flap and it is also dangerous to do so.
13. *Flap inset (Fig. 9.32.2):* After confirming the hemostasis and the viability of the flap, inset can be done with 4.0 Ethilon using half buried horizontal mattress suturing.
14. *Management of the donor area:* After confirming hemostasis, the residual raw area on the middle finger should be covered with a split thickness skin graft. At the points where the defect crosses the proximal interphalangeal (PIP) and distal interphalangeal (DIP) joint creases, back cuts should be given for 3 mm to avoid skin graft contractures later on. Now, raise the hand and prepare the arm with betadine solution. The skin graft should be harvested from the medial side of the arm. Sterile dressings should be applied over the skin graft donor site before moving back to the hand. The graft should be applied over the raw area and tie over sutures applied with 3.0 Ethilon.
15. Sterile dressings should be applied over the hand and the forearm. Care must

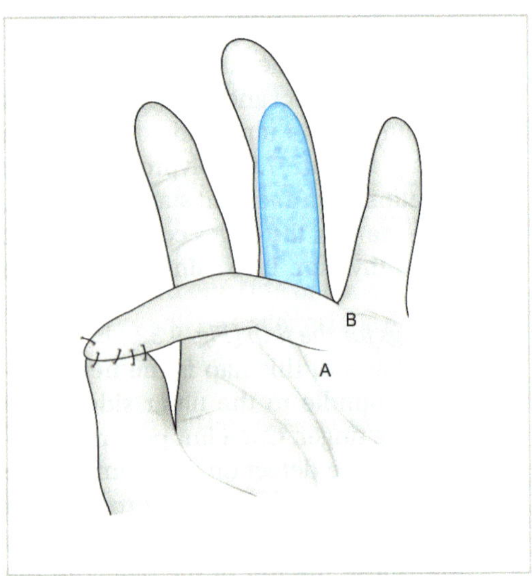

Fig. 9.32.2 After final flap inset

be taken to avoid compression of the pedicle at any point of its course. A finger dressing must be applied on the middle finger. A sterile gauze must be placed under the flap which is bridging the base of the middle finger with the stump of the thumb. A dorsal POP slab should be applied for the thumb keeping the wrist in neutral, and the MCP joint of the thumb in flexion of 20° and interphalangeal (IP) joints in extension. A window must be made in the dressings to allow inspection and monitoring of the flap.

Postoperative Protocol

- Admission in the ward
- The affected hand should be kept elevated
- Patient can take normal diet immediately if the procedure was under regional block or after complete recovery if under general anesthesia
- Clinical monitoring of the flap once every 6 hours
- Analgesics and antibiotics for 5 days
- Sedation SOS for 1 day
- Inspection of the dressing after 48 hours
- Discharge of the patient by third day
- Suture removal on the 10th day and removal of donor site dressing on the arm
- Removal of the POP slabs on the 14th day and execute the second stage of surgery.

Stage II

1. The preferred anesthesia is either axillary block or general anesthesia (in children)
2. Apply the tourniquet and keep ready
3. Preparation and draping as described in Appendix I. The elbow area must also be prepared and kept exposed
4. Raise the tourniquet and note the time
5. Divide the base of the flap close to the place where it is attached to the middle finger. The digital vessel to the middle finger will now be cut and must be ligated
6. The stump of the flap must now be sutured to the skin grafted edge on the middle finger
7. On the thumb, through the exposure provided by the divided flap, the stump of the ulnar side digital nerve to the thumb must be identified and dissected. Since surgeons have already tagged this nerve end with 7.0 polypropylene suture materials, it may be easily identifiable. Now, on the cut edge of the flap, the digital vessel must be ligated. The cut end of the digital nerve entering the flap is now dissected for about 2 to 3 mm, to allow for nerve coaptation
8. The two nerve ends are coapted with 7.0 polypropylenes
9. The tourniquet is released and hemostasis is achieved
10. The final inset is now done with 4.0 Ethilon. Sterile dressings are done and a thumb dressing is provided.

Postoperative Protocol

- Patient can be treated as an outpatient
- The affected hand should be kept elevated
- Patient can take normal diet immediately if the procedure was under regional block or after complete recovery if under general anesthesia
- Analgesics and antibiotics for 5 days
- Sedation SOS for 1 day
- Inspection of the dressing after 48 hours
- Suture removal on the 10th day. Refer to physiotherapy for active and passive mobilization of the fingers and thumb
- Daily wash with soap and water
- Massage of scar and grafted skin with coconut oil
- Compression garment for scar softening after a further 2 weeks.

Procedures for Reconstruction of Type III Amputations

33

Osteoplastic Reconstruction

One of the methods of staged reconstruction of a thumb that has been amputated at the level between the neck of the proximal phalanx and the metacarpophalangeal (MCP) joint (type III amputation) is the osteoplastic reconstruction.

The requirements for a thumb amputated at this level are:

- To provide length with soft tissues and skin cover
- To provide stability with bone
- To provide sensation on the pulp region of the reconstructed thumb
- To provide for the lost movement at the lost interphalangeal (IP) joint region
- To provide for good cosmetic appearance with a nail complex.

However, the method of reconstruction that surgeons are going to consider now, does not provide all the above. However, this method of reconstruction has its own advantages.

Advantages

- A relatively simple method of reconstruction and does not require microsurgical skills
- Provides adequate length to the thumb
- Excellent stability is provided by the use of the bone graft
- Preserves the already available movement at the carpometacarpal (CMC) joint, and hence, coarse movements of the thumb are preserved
- Provides good sensation on the tip and pulp – provided by the Littler's neurovascular Island flap component of this method of reconstruction.

Disadvantages

- Does not provide the lost movement at the level of an IP joint
- Is a staged procedure and hence, takes time
- Does not provide cosmesis, as the nail complex is not restored.

The components of this method of reconstruction are as follows:

- Stage I: Tubed groin flap to augment the length with a skin envelope followed by division and inset of the flap
- Stage II: Free bone graft to provide stability to the skin tube
- Littler's neurovascular Island flap to provide sensation to the tip and pulp of the reconstructed thumb.

Surgical Steps

1. Component I: Tubed groin flap
2. Component II: Ulnar bone graft application
3. Component III: Littler's neurovascular Island flap

Surgical Procedure of Component I (Tubed Groin Flap)

1. Debridement of the hand wound can be done under axillary block anesthesia and spinal anesthesia or tumescent local

anesthetic for raising the flap. In children, general anesthesia may be used.

2. The patient should be placed in a supine position. A rolled up towel should be placed under the gluteal region on the side that the flap is going to be raised. This position makes raising the flap easy.
3. Now, the groin region is prepared, from the subcostal margin to the groin region and from the midline to the mid-axillary line on the same side of the injured hand. If the flap planned is large, the ipsilateral thigh is also prepared. The hand is also prepared and draped.
4. Now, debridement of the hand wound is done. After debriding the wound, a lint pattern is taken of the defect on the hand. The tourniquet is released and hemostasis is achieved. The tourniquet is removed and the site of application on the arm is massaged by the theater assistant.
5. Markings are now made on the groin region. The first marking is the anterior superior iliac spine. Next the pubic tubercle is marked. These two points are joined by a curvilinear line convex downward. The femoral artery is palpated and marked for about 3 cm from the inguinal ligament distally. Now, a point is marked on this femoral artery line, about 2.5 cm (2 finger breadths) distal to the inguinal ligament. Another point is marked 2.5 cm (2 finger breadths) lateral to this point. This point is where the axial artery of the flap-superficial circumflex iliac artery enters the flap. Now, draw a line from this point parallel to the inguinal ligament up to the anterior superior iliac spine. This is the course of this artery.
6. Place the lint pattern of the defect with the pedicle at the marked pivot point of the flap. The flap can be marked with equal breadth superior and inferior to the axis of the flap. When the flap extends beyond the anterior superior iliac spine, it has restricted dimensions. If, at the level of the anterior superior iliac spine, the width of the flap is 6 cm, the flap can only extend for 6 cm beyond the anterior superior iliac spine. This is because this portion of the flap is a random portion and must follow the 1:1 ratio. The flap is now marked following the above principles.
7. The first incision is made on the distal portion of the flap with a number 22 blade down to the skin, subcutaneous tissue up to fascia. Incision is then made on the superior margin up to the membranous layer of the superficial fascia. The inferior incision is made up to the deep fascia. Now, incisions have been completed on 3 sides. By placing two skin hooks on the distal portion of the flap, and applying gentle traction, the flap is raised from the bed in the plane of loose areolar tissue superficial to the deep fascia. The flap is raised thus till the marked pivot point. The viability of the flap can be confirmed by noting the bleeding from the edges of the flap.
8. The donor site of the flap should now be covered. If it is small, it can be closed primarily in layers, with 2.0 Vicryl subcutaneous sutures, and 3.0 polypropylenes for skin. This can be facilitated by flexing at the hip to ease the suture line till closure of the skin. If the defect is large, it should first be narrowed by suturing the edge of the skin to the deep fascia with 3.0 Vicryl and making the residual raw area smaller. The residual raw area should then be covered with a split thickness skin graft harvested from the thigh. The donor site of the graft should be covered with vaseline gauze and dressing with pads and bandage. The skin graft should be applied on the raw area in the groin and anchored with 3.0 silk. Sterile vaseline gauze and pad is applied.
9. Now, the hand is brought to the groin region and insetting of the flap is done, i.e. the suturing of the flap to the edges of the defect. This is done with 3.0 polyamide suture material.
10. After the flap inset is done, vaseline gauze is applied over the suture line. Arm and

elbow restraints are applied with pad and sticking plaster, to maintain the position of the hand in a comfortable position for the patient.

Stage of flap division: This is done on Day 14.

- Local anesthetic or tumescent solution is injected in the base of the flap. It is then incised with a number 15 blade and the hand separated from the groin region
- Hemostasis is achieved and the groin wound is closed with 3.0 polypropylene sutures. Sterile dressings are applied on the groin and hand wound.

Stage of final flap inset: This is done on Day 16 (2 days after flap division)

- Axillary block anesthesia is given
- The hand is painted and draped. The flap edges are looked for necrosis. Any necrosed portion is excised. If there is no necrosis the flap edge is trimmed for about 3 mm.

Suturing this edge to the edge of the defect is done with 3.0 polyamide suture. Sterile dressings are done.

After a period of about 3 months which is needed for the skin flap to become soft and supple and the joint of thumb to become active again (after the period of immobilization in the groin flap), the second stage of the reconstruction is done. This comprises of two components, both done in the same stage.

Surgical Procedure of Component II (Ulnar Bone Graft Application)

- Preparation and draping are done as described in Appendix I.
- The scar on the volar aspect of the groin flap skin is excised and the volar seam line of the groin flap is opened. This will expose the stump of the bone, which may be either the base of the proximal phalanx or the head of the metacarpal bone. The exposed stump of bone must be freshened by nibbling away the sclerotic layer. If the remaining base of the proximal phalanx is very small (less than 0.5 cm), it can be excised.
- Now, a hole must be drilled in the end of the bone to receive the bone graft. This is because, the ulnar bone graft which is a corticocancellous graft is going to be used and the most effective method of fixation would be to peg the bone graft into a hole in the stump of bone.
- The procedure of harvesting the ulnar bone graft is described in the Appendix VI.

Surgical Procedure of Component III (Littler's Neurovascular Island Flap)

Once the bone graft has been pegged into place, the opening that was made in the volar aspect of the groin flap must be resurfaced with the neurovascular flap. The defect is measured and the neurovascular Island flap done as described in chapter 3.

Postoperative Protocol

- Admission in the ward
- The affected hand should be kept elevated
- Patient can take normal diet immediately if the procedure was under regional block or after complete recovery if under general anesthesia
- Clinical monitoring of the flap once every 6 hours
- Analgesics and antibiotics for 5 days
- Sedation sos for 1 day
- Inspection of the dressing after 48 hours
- Discharge of the patient by third day
- Suture removal on the 10th day and removal of donor site dressing on the arm
- Removal of the POP slab on the 14 day and advise the following:
    - Refer to physiotherapy for active and passive mobilization of the fingers and thumb
    - Daily wash with soap and water
    - Massage of scar and grafted skin with coconut oil
    - Compression garment for scar softening after a further 2 weeks
    - Straightening splint for the middle finger to be worn for 3 weeks at night.

Vascularized Wrap-around Great Toe Transfer

Preparation

- Palpate the dorsalis pedis artery, Doppler it and mark the course.
- Put the leg in a dependent position and mark the main dorsal veins, the transverse arch and the great saphenous system.
- Measure the circumference of the normal thumb at the level of the MCP joint. Measure the circumference of the ipsilateral great toe at the metatarsophalangeal (MTP) joint.
- Measure the length of the normal thumb and the length of the thumb to be reconstructed. The difference between the two values will give the measurement of the ipsilateral great toe required as a flap (Fig. 9.33.1). The difference between the two values represents the width of the flap of skin on the medial side of the great toe. This flap is marked on the medial side of the great toe and this flap extends distally to the tip of the great toe with a tapering tip.
- Next, the marking of the flap (Fig. 9.33.2) is made. If the circumference of the thumb is 7.5 cm, a 7.5 cm circumferential line is drawn at the base of the ipsilateral great toe. Now, the medial flap must be outlined, which is necessary to protect the remaining portion of the great toe. A line is drawn on the dorsum of the great toe from the tip to the circumferential base line on the medial side including the medial nail fold. From the medial eponychium, this line is extended laterally, about 2 to 3 mm beneath the nail. A similar line is marked on the plantar aspect of the great toe to meet the above line at the level of the lateral toe tip.
- Mark a point "A" at the level of the distal edge of the inferior extensor retinaculum, halfway between the dorsalis pedis artery marking and the great saphenous system marking.
- Draw an "S" shaped line between the point "A" and the marked circumferential base line adjacent to the first web space.

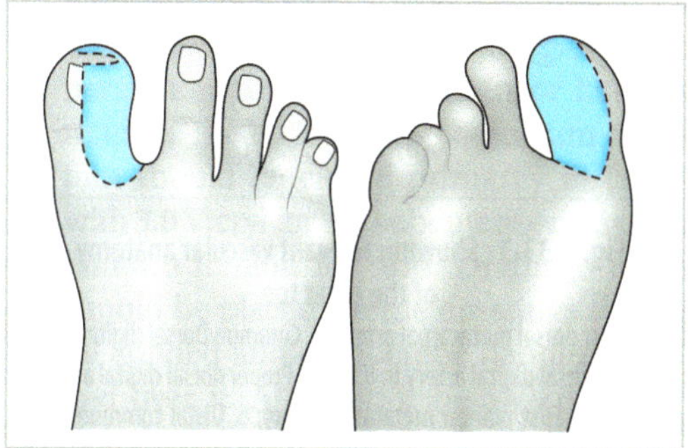

Fig. 9.33.1 Showing the amount of skin on the great toe to be harvested as a flap

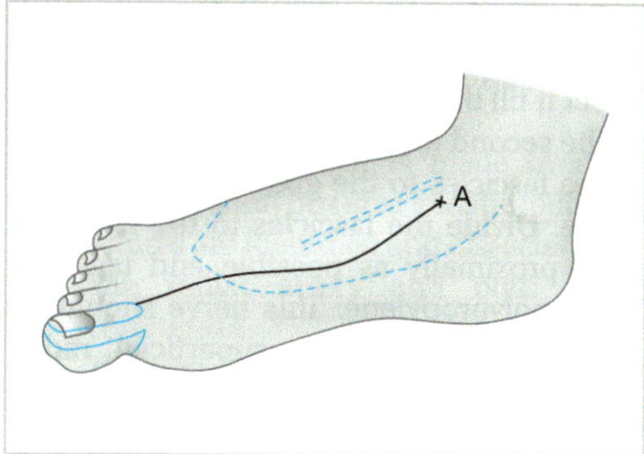

Fig. 9.33.2 Marking for the dissection of the pedicle

Surgical Steps

1. Prepare the ipsilateral lower limb from the knee distally and apply the drapings.
2. The tourniquet can be raised and the time noted.
3. Make the dorsal incision down to the dermis only.
4. Raise medial and lateral flaps for about 2 to 3 cm on either side.
5. The following should be dissected now - the great saphenous vein, other dorsal veins, fat and subcutaneous tissue.
6. Dissect the dorsalis pedis artery up to the distal part of the intermetatarsal space, where it will divide into two branches to the great toe and the second toe.

the shape of a "cricket bat", to enable the "handle" end to be pegged into the head of the metacarpal bone. Place the bone graft in normal saline

- Close the donor site of the bone graft in layers with 3.0 Vicryl for the subcutaneous tissues and 4.0 Ethilon for skin. Drainage tubes should be placed. Sterile dressings should be applied
- Now, peg the bone graft into the stump of the bone that has been prepared. This must be done in such a way that the cancellous side faces the dorsal aspect
- Apply gentle compression with moist gauze and padding over the wound. Release the tourniquet. Hold the hand in an elevated position for a period of 4 to 5 minutes. Rest the hand on the table and secure hemostasis.

Fixation of the Toe Flap

- Bring the wrap around great toe flap to the recipient site. Place the toe over the pegged bone graft and get a good position, a position in which good opposition can be achieved with the fingers and is a functional position
- A subcutaneous tunnel is created between the recipient site vessels and the summit of the stump. This tunnel is for the vessels of the toe to be passed through to reach the recipient vessels—the radial artery
- The structures to be passed through the tunnel are:
    - The arteries
    - The veins
    - The deep peroneal nerve.
- Nerve repair—the digital nerves are sutured to the two plantar digital nerves of the toe and the deep peroneal nerve is sutured to the superficial branch of the radial nerve at the anatomical snuff box. The nerve repairs are done with 7.0 polypropylene using epineurial sutures
- Vascular anastomosis—the recipient vessels should be divided, blood flow checked from the divided artery and approximator clamps applied. The soft clamps must be released from the donor vessels. Vascular anastomosis should be done (the technique of vascular anastomosis is beyond the scope of this manual).
- Bulky sterile dressings and above elbow POP are applied with the elbow in 90° flexion, forearm in mid prone position. A bulky dressing is applied on the leg and foot with a posterior below knee POP slab.

Postoperative Protocol

- Admission in the ward
- The affected hand and the donor foot should be kept elevated
- Patient is kept on nil oral for 24 hours in case of need for exploration if there is a vascular problem in the flap
- Clinical monitoring of the flap once every hour
- Analgesics and antibiotics for 5 days
- Sedation SOS for 1 day
- Inspection of the dressing after 48 hours
- Suture removal on the 10th day
- Removal of the POP slab on the 21st day. If across toe flap has been done for coverage of the donor site, the flap has to be divided at this time
- Refer to physiotherapy for active and passive mobilization of the fingers and thumb
- Daily wash with soap and water
- Massage of scar and grafted skin with coconut oil
- Compression garment for scar softening after a further 2 weeks.

Procedures for Reconstruction of Type IV Amputations

34

Vascularized Second Toe Transfer

Preparation

- Palpate the dorsalis pedis artery and mark the course
- Put the leg in a dependent position and mark the main dorsal veins, the transverse arch and the great saphenous system
- Mark a dorsal triangle on the dorsum of the foot (Fig. 9.34.1) 2 cm length and 1 cm base at the second toe. Mark the plantar triangle about 1.5 cm and 1.0 cm (in adults, this triangle measures 4 cm by 2.5 cm on the dorsum and 3 cm by 2 cm)
- Mark a point "A" at the level of the distal edge of the inferior extensor retinaculum, halfway between the dorsalis pedis artery marking and the great saphenous system marking
- Draw a curvilinear line between the point "A" and the apex of the marked triangle
- Similarly, from the apex of the triangle on the plantar aspect, make a marking that extends from the apex proximally along the second metatarsal to the midsole.

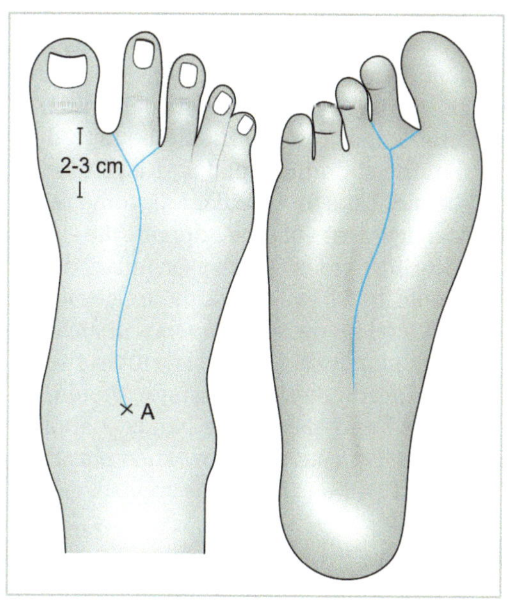

Fig. 9.34.1 Markings for the second toe harvest

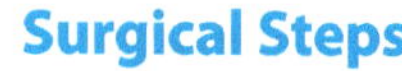

Surgical Steps

1. Make the dorsal incision down to the dermis only.
2. Raise medial and lateral flaps for about 2 to 3 cm on either side.
3. The following should be dissected now – the great saphenous vein, other dorsal veins, fat and subcutaneous tissue.
4. Dissect the dorsalis pedis artery up to the distal part of the intermetatarsal space, where it will divide into two branches to the great toe and the second toe.
5. Dissect the deep peroneal nerve which lies deep to the dorsalis pedis artery. Dissect it till the divisions to the great toe and the second toe. Tease gently and separate the fascicles to the great toe and second toe. Divide the fascicles to the second toe as proximally as possible and tagged with 7.0 polypropylenes.

6. Dissect the extensor hallucis longus tendon and divide it at the level of the distal edge of the inferior extensor retinaculum. Divide the tendon of the extensor brevis at the level of the metatarsal base.
7. At the distal part of the dorsalis pedis artery, identify the deep communicating branch going to the plantar side. This branch will join with the first plantar metatarsal artery to form the plantar digital artery. And this plantar digital artery will divide into two, the medial plantar digital artery going to the lateral side of great toe and the lateral plantar digital artery going to the second toe. Examine this system to see which is dominant—the first dorsal metatarsal artery and the dorsal digital arteries or the first plantar metatarsal arteries and the plantar digital arteries.
8. Now, surgeons go to the plantar side dissection. Make the plantar incisions. The medial and lateral plantar digital nerves are identified. The fascicles to the great toe and the fascicles to the third toe teased from the medial and plantar digital nerves respectively. The fascicles going to the second toe are cut as proximal as possible and tagged with 7.0 polypropylenes.
9. The flexor digitorum brevis muscle is cut at the midsole level, where it joins the tendon of the long flexor. The long flexor tendon is divided at the midsole level.
10. The medial plantar digital artery (branch to the great toe) is divided.
11. The transverse metatarsal ligament is divided on the medial and lateral aspect of the metatarsophalangeal (MTP) joint of the second toe. Great care should be taken at this level to avoid injury to the vessels at this level.
12. Now, retractors should be applied to the second metatarsal and retracted laterally and the first metatarsal retracted medially. The arterial system is now exposed. The system should be carefully dissected, taking into account the dominance of the vessel system. This can be assisted by carefully dividing the interosseous muscles and further exposing the arterial system.
13. Now, the second toe is almost completely dissected and is held only by the intact metatarsal bone and the artery and veins. The osteotomy of the metatarsal can be done. This should be done depending on the length that surgeons have already calculated in the preoperative work-up.
14. Once the osteotomy is over, the remaining soft tissues can be divided, so that the second toe is now held only by the arteries and veins.
15. Now, release the tourniquet, apply warm, moist pads over the second toe and the vascular pedicle. Take care to prevent the toe from falling down and shearing the vessels. Raise the foot for about 5 minutes. Then place the foot on the table. It usually takes about 15 to 20 minutes for the circulation to be re-established in the dissected toe. By the end of this time, the toe becomes pink and warm and ready for transfer.
16. The vessels can be divided when the recipient site dissection is over.
17. Division of the pedicle—soft clamps should be applied over the artery and veins. The proximal ends of the artery and veins should be ligated with 3.0 Vicryl. The vessels should be divided and the time noted. The flap should be placed on a moist abdominal pad and taken to the recipient site for vascular anastomosis.
18. Management of the donor site—after securing hemostasis, the secondary defect should be closed primarily in layers with 3.0 Vicryl for the subcutaneous tissues and 4.0 Ethilon for skin. Drainage tubes should be placed. Sterile dressings should be applied and elastocrépe bandage applied over it. A posterior below knee plaster of Paris (POP) slab should be applied.

Recipient Site Dissection

- The hand is prepared as described in Appendix I

- A curvilinear incision is made over the anatomical snuffbox area and the following structures are identified and dissected:
  - The radial artery and both venae comitantes
  - The cephalic vein
  - The superficial branch of the radial nerve.
- One percent of Xylocaine gauze is applied over the dissected vessels
- A volar incision is made on the stump of the thumb proximally up to the thenar area. Raise the medial and lateral skin flaps, apply anchoring sutures with 3.0 Ethilon and dissect the following structures:
  - The flexor pollicis longus tendon
  - The digital nerves—the ends should be tagged with 7.0 polypropylene
  - The extensor pollicis longus tendon
  - Prepare the end of the bony stump to which the second toe is going to be fixed.
- Apply gentle compression with moist gauze and padding over the wound. Release the tourniquet. Hold the hand in an elevated position for a period of 4 ot 5 minutes. Rest the hand on the table and secure hemostasis.

Fixation of the Toe Flap

- Bring the toe flap to the recipient site. Place the toe over the stump and get a good position, a position in which good opposition can be achieved with the fingers and is a functional position.
- A subcutaneous tunnel is created between the recipient site vessels and the summit of the stump. This tunnel is for the vessels of the toe to be passed through to reach the recipient vessels—the radial artery.
- The structures to be passed through the tunnel are:
  - The arteries
  - The veins
  - The deep peroneal nerve.
- *Bone fixation*—is done with K-wires without causing damage to the vessels.
- *Tendon repair*—the flexor longus tendon of the toe is sutured to the flexor pollicis longus tendon end and the extensor longus tendon of the toe is sutured to the end of the extensor pollicis longus tendon. The tension should be adjusted, so that, the toe is stable and in a functional position. The repair is done with 3.0 polypropylenes using modified KM suture technique.
- *Nerve repair*—the digital nerves are sutured to the two plantar digital nerves of the toe and the deep peroneal nerve is sutured to the superficial branch of the radial nerve at the anatomical snuff box. The nerve repairs are done with 7.0 polypropylene using epineurial sutures.
- *Joint repair*—the MTP joint of the toe is primarily in a position of hyperextension. When this toe is transferred to become a thumb, if it retains this position, the reconstructed thumb may not be functional as it may be away from the fingers. So, it is important that the MTP joint be made more physiological. To do this, the volar capsule of the MTP joint is plicated with 4.0 polypropylenes.
- *Vascular anastomosis*—the recipient vessels should be divided, blood flow checked from the divided artery and approximator clamps applied. The soft clamps must be released from the donor vessels. Vascular anastomosis should be done (the technique of vascular anastomosis is beyond the scope of this manual).
- Bulky sterile dressings and above elbow POP are applied with the elbow in 90° flexion, forearm in mid prone position. A bulky dressing is applied on the leg and foot with a posterior below knee POP slab.

Postoperative Protocol

- Admission in the ward
- The affected hand and the donor foot should be kept elevated
- Patient is kept on nil oral for 24 hours in case of need for exploration if there is a vascular problem in the flap
- Clinical monitoring of the flap once every hour

- Analgesics and antibiotics for 5 days
- Sedation SOS for 1 day
- Inspection of the dressing after 48 hours
- Suture removal on the 10th day
- Removal of the POP slab on the 21st day. If across toe flap has been done for coverage of the donor site, the flap has to be divided at this time
- Refer to physiotherapy for active and passive mobilization of the fingers and thumb
- Daily wash with soap and water
- Massage of scar and grafted skin with coconut oil
- Compression garment for scar softening after a further 2 weeks.

Procedures for Reconstruction of Type V Amputations

35

Pollicization

Presurgical Counseling

- This procedure will be done under axillary block anesthesia or general anesthesia
- The procedure consists of harvesting a tendon graft from the index finger. There will be no deficit on the index finger as a result of this
- This procedure will take about 1½ to 2 hours to perform
- A dressing will be applied and a plaster of Paris (POP) slab will be applied at the end of surgery
- Admission will be necessary for a minimum period of 3 days
- Postoperatively, no movements of the fingers should be attempted. If it is done, the sutured tendons may rupture
- Postoperatively, the POP slab will be continued for a period of 3 weeks. After this period, physiotherapy will be started and this should be done for another 3 weeks
- In some instances, even if the movements of the finger improve, further surgery may be required to release the scars that may form
- The general complications of anesthetic infiltration like hypersensitivity may occur in spite of test dose application. This complication will cause dryness of mouth and apprehension, which can be corrected immediately.

Surgical Steps

Described in Chapter on Hypoplastic thump pollicization.

SECTION

10

Tumors

Ganglion Excision

36

Introduction

One of the most common tumors occurring on the hand is the ganglion, which can occur on the volar side or the dorsal aspect of the wrist. The surgical management of both these conditions is described here.

Salient Features of the Condition

1. Is believed to occur due to degenerative changes in the joint capsule.
2. Is prone for recurrence after surgery due to incomplete removal of the intra-articular portion of the ganglion.
3. Complete removal and prevention of recurrence is dependent on following the principles of hand surgery, i.e. regional block anesthesia (axillary or supraclavicular block), use of tourniquet, use of magnification, bipolar cautery and a liberal incision to expose and excise the tumor.

The surgical steps for the excision of volar and dorsal ganglions are the same and they are discussed here.

Surgical Steps

1. Apply a pneumatic tourniquet on the upper arm.
2. Prepare and drape the involved upper limb from the elbow to the tip of the hand.
3. Mark a transverse incision over the summit of the tumor (volar or dorsal). The incision should extend beyond the circumference of the tumor by about 3 to 4 mm.
4. Raise the tourniquet.
5. Make the incision as marked down through the dermis.
6. Apply skin hooks on one of the edges and lift the skin flap off the surface of the ganglion. Elevate this flap till the corresponding edge of the ganglion is visible. Repeat this procedure on the opposite edge of the flap. So, now the entire circumference of the ganglion will be visible on retracting both skin edges.
7. The ganglion will have a narrow stalk as it arises from the intra-articular area. This must be dissected by gently elevating the circumference of the ganglion from the bed, formed by the surface of the joint capsule. The points to be noted when doing this step are:
    - The tendons on either side should be retracted carefully to the radial and ulnar sides to avoid injury to them
    - The ganglion should not be grasped with forceps as this may injure the wall of the ganglion and lead to leak of the mucoid material. The method of retracting the ganglion is by either retaining some soft tissues over the surface to enable surgeons to hold it, or by atraumatic retraction with a piece of saline gauze

- In the case of volar ganglion, the radial artery and its venae comitantes may course close to the edge of the tumor. Care should be exercised to avoid injury to these vessels by appropriate retraction.

8. Once the ganglion has been raised off the surface of the joint capsule, and the extension into the joint identified, an incision must be made on the joint capsule up to the edge of the ganglion stalk and the intra-articular area exposed. By this incision, the stalk of the ganglion can be traced over the articular surfaces of the carpal bones down to the intercarpal ligaments.
9. The entire stalk of the ganglion can be removed by gentle blunt dissection to free it from the intercarpal ligament. Thus, the entire ganglion can be excised in-toto.
10. The tourniquet should be released and hemostasis achieved. The rent in the joint capsule should not be closed. A Segmüller drain (tubing of the scalp vein set) kept and the wound closed in layers with 4.0 Vicryl for the subcutaneous tissues and skin closed with 3.0 polypropylene subcuticular sutures, with the drainage tube coming out from one end of the suture line. Non-adherent dressings applied and plaster of Paris (POP) slab should be applied to immobilize the wrist. For the dorsal ganglion, a volar POP slab should be applied with the wrist in 20° extension, and for the volar ganglion, a dorsal POP slab should be applied with the wrist in 10° flexion.

Postoperative Protocol

- The patient may be treated as an outpatient with the advise to keep the hand elevated, oral antibiotics for 3 days, analgesics and anti-inflammatory agents
- The suture line must be examined at the end of 48 hours and the drainage tube removed. Dressings must be applied again and the POP slab retained
- On the 10th day, the suture can be removed, and the POP slab removed
- Patient may be advised the following:
  - Wash with soap and water
  - Scar massage with coconut oil
  - Active and passive movements of the wrist and fingers at physiotherapy
  - Compression garment after 2 weeks to soften the scar, to be worn for a minimum of 3 weeks.

SECTION

11

Degenerative Conditions

Dupuytren's Contracture—Assessment

37

Introduction

Dupuytren's contracture is a relatively uncommon condition that surgeons see in the outpatient department in South India, but when a patient does present, management should be perfect to relieve the patient of his distress and make his hand a useful one.

The points to be noted in the assessment are described below:

History

- History of diabetes mellitus, alcohol intake or epilepsy, or family history of the disorder. These are important findings not only for the diagnosis of the problem, but also to prognosticate the results
- Though patients with diabetes present mainly with a mild form of the disease consisting of palmar nodules, the rate of recurrence after surgical management of contractures, if they develop, are quite high
- Similarly, patients who give history of alcohol intake are also prone for complications after surgical management of Dupuytren's disease
- Eliciting a history of trauma, however trivial, may also be significant, because, in such situations, the prognosis is very good and recurrence rates are very minimal.

Symptoms

- Tightness in the palm on extension
- Nodules or callus like formation in the palm
- Gradually increasing contracture of the fingers
- Maceration of skin within contracture folds and secondary infection.

Clinical Examination

- *Nodules*—usually present in the area of the distal palm particularly at the level of the palmar creases. Usually non-tender and painless
- *Skin pits*—are sometimes seen in the plamar region
- Sometimes, there is just a distortion of the palmar creases; either deepening of the creases or widening of the creases. These are significant, since they denote the early stages of the disease. However, it is not essential for these lesions to progress and lead to contractures
    - *Palpable cords*—different types of cord formation which lead to different types of contractures and need different surgical management plans. If the cord is palpable, the extent of the cord should be noted

- Sometimes, even the neurovascular bundles on either side of thickened cords may be palpable as soft fluffy swellings, especially when they are deformed by the spiraling cords
- *Contractures*—when there is a minimal contracture, the easy way to find it is to ask the patient to place the palm of the hand flat on the surface of the table. This will not be possible even in mild contractures of the metacarpophalangeal (MCP) joint. The contractures in the MCP joint, proximal interphalangeal (PIP) joint and the distal interphalangeal (DIP) joint should be noted. The passive and active range of movements in these joints should also be recorded. The angle of the contracture is also noted and will help to classify the deformity according to the Tubiana-Michon system. The method of recording is to measure the contracture angle from the neutral line and add up the values of the contractures on the MCP and PIP joints. This is applicable for fingers and thumb
- *Secondary problems of contractures*—like skin maceration, deformities of the nail complexes should be noted.

Staging

Staging of Dupuytren's contracture—assessment are given in Table 11.37.1.

Table 11.37.1 Staging of Dupuytren's contracture—assessment

Contractures	*Description*	*Stage*
Nil		0
< 45°		I
45°–90°	MCP contracture > PIP contracture	II
	PIP contracture > MCP contracture	II D
90°–135°	MCP contracture > PIP contracture	III
	PIP contracture > MCP contracture	III D
> 135°	MCP contracture > PIP contracture	IV
	PIP contracture > MCP contracture	IV D

Planning the Management

Planning of management of Dupuytren's contracture—assessment are given in Table 11.37.2.

Table 11.37.2 Planning of management of Dupuytren's contracture—assessment

Findings	*Plan*
Stage 0: Only nodules or pits	Conservative management Stretching exercises, local steroid injection
Stage I	No surgery required unless patient requests
Stage II: Only one or two rays	Fasciectomy
Stage II: Multiple rays Stage III	Open palm technique/ fasciectomy
Stage IV	Distractor application before fasciectomy

Planning the Timing of the Surgery

When the contracture involves only the MCP joint, the surgery need not be done immediately as there is no risk of involvement of the joint. However, in cases of mainly PIP joint, it is important to schedule the surgery as early as possible to avoid irreversible contracture of the joint.

Dupuytren's Contracture—Management

38

Fasciectomy

Surgical Steps

- Prepare the hand as described in Appendix I
- Marking the incisions (Fig. 11.38.1):
    - The zig-zag incisions of Bruner are marked on the palm and affected finger rays, beginning proximally from the hollow of the palm between the thenar and hypothenar eminences. The incisions follow the course of the flexor tendons of each finger.

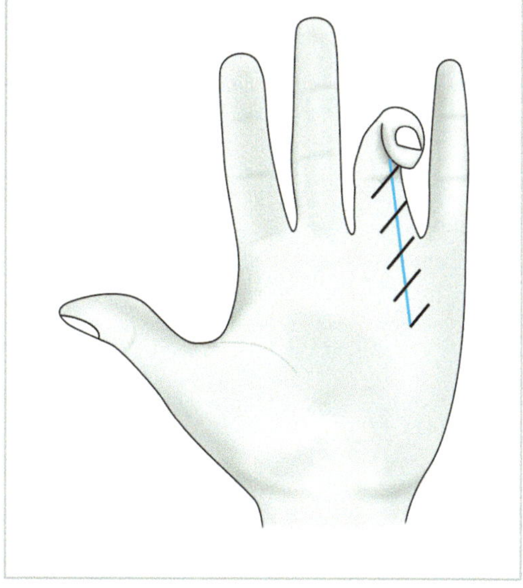

Fig. 11.38.1 Marking the incisions for fasciectomy

- The tourniquet is raised and the incisions are made
- The incision is made down through the skin and subcutaneous tissues only and the skin flaps are raised on either side
- The contracted and thickened fascia is carefully dissected and isolated. It is very important to keep the neurovascular bundles in sight throughout the dissection procedure. This is to avoid inadvertent injury to the neurovascular bundles
- Once the entire length of the fascia is dissected, it is excised
- Moist saline gauze pieces are placed over the wound and the hand is raised. Gentle compression is applied over the gauze. The tourniquet is released and the compression is maintained for 3 minutes. The hand is then placed back on the table and hemostasis is secured. The viability of the skin flaps is confirmed
- Suturing of the wounds is done with 4.0 Ethilon, after keeping Segmüller drainage tubes
- Sterile dressings are applied and a dorsal plaster of Paris (POP) slab is applied with the wrist in 30° extension, metacarpophalangeal (MCP) joints of fingers in 40° flexion and interphalangeal (IP) joints of the fingers kept straight.

Postoperative Protocol

- Admission in the ward
- The affected hand should be kept elevated

- Patient can take normal diet immediately if the procedure was under regional block or after complete recovery if under general anesthesia
- Inspection of the suture line after 48 hours without disturbing the position of the POP slab
- Discharge of the patient by third day
- Suture removal on the 10th day
- Plaster of Paris is also removed on the 10th day
- Advise the following:
    - Refer to physiotherapy for active mobilization of the fingers
    - Daily wash with soap and water
    - Massage of scar and grafted skin with coconut oil
- Application of a detachable straightening splint for the affected fingers throughout the day for 3 weeks. Intermittently, the splint should be removed and active and passive mobilization of fingers should be done. The splint should be worn for another 3 weeks at night
- The unaffected fingers should be mobilized from the day of POP removal
- Patient is advised to continue the mobilization of the fingers; both active and passive and review once every month for evaluation.
- It is practical to advise the patient to carry a brief case or portfolio, which keeps the MCP joints in extended position and stretched to the maximum.

SECTION

12

Infection

Hansen's Disease and Sequelae

39

History

- Duration of complaints—will indicate the progress of the lesion
- History of treatment—both medical and surgical
- Occupation of the patient—this is important for deciding the surgical reconstruction
- A patient who does manual labor will need powerful tendon transfers, while patients doing sedentary type of labor will require the transfer of less powerful muscles. In such patients, even static procedures will sometimes suffice
- Episodes of drug reactions—a history of lepra reaction and the time of the reaction will be important in deciding the timing of surgical reconstruction.

Clinical Examination

Type of Hand

Some people have soft hands with hypermobile joints. The force required to move these joints is very little, as the joints are very supple and the skin and soft tissues are also very supple. Hence, when tendon transfers are planned for such patients, care should be exercised in choosing the donor tendon [avoid removing the flexor digitorum superficialis (FDS) of the finger] and in choosing the type of tendon transfer (avoid using powerful tendon transfers like Brand's procedure). Procedures like Fowler's procedure may well suit such patients. On the other hand, patients with bulky hands with thickened skin will require more powerful transfers.

Attitude of the Hand

The following positions of the hand may be seen:

- Total claw of the hand—the metacarpophalangeal (MCP) joints are hyperextended, interphalangeal (IP) joints are flexed in all the fingers. This signifies combined low ulnar and median nerve palsy
- Ulnar fingers alone in clawed position—may denote that there is a low ulnar nerve palsy. However, the involvement of the median nerve also cannot be ruled out
- Fingers in cascade but the thumb is lying in the plane of the palm—denotes the involvement of the median nerve at the level of the distal forearm
- Fingers appear to be in cascade—ask the patient to extend all the fingers. This will show the claw if it is present
- Thumb and index finger are kept extended, while the other fingers are in cascade—will indicate a high level median nerve lesion
- All the fingers, thumb and the wrist are in flexed position, with inability to extend any of them—indicates a radial nerve lesion
- "Z" deformity of the thumb indicates a combined low median and ulnar palsy
- A flat palm, with the metacarpal arch obliteration points to the combined low median and ulnar nerve palsy.

Appearance of the Hand

- Skin appears shiny and bereft of skin ridges—indicates a combined median and ulnar nerve lesion
- Absorption of the fingertip and deformities of the nail will denote long standing disease
- Wasting of the thenar eminence on the palm—indicates a median nerve lesion. This lesion can be either low level or high level lesion
- Wasting of the hypothenar eminence indicates an ulnar nerve lesion
- Hollowing of the intermetacarpal spaces on the dorsum of the hand also signifies ulnar nerve lesion
- Presence of ulcers—are significant and usually found on typical areas like over the heads of the metacarpals, tips of the fingers, and on the volar aspect of the wrist
- Presence of scars—may indicate healed ulcers. In some patients, scars may give a clue about the previously done reconstructive procedures, if any.

By now, there will be a clue about which nerve has been involved in the disease process. So, the next step consists of testing the individual nerve territory separately for the three nerves. There are many standard tests described in textbooks, and a few of them are mentioned here.

For the Ulnar Nerve

Ulnar nerve of Hansen's disease and sequelae are shown in Table 12.39.1.

For the Median Nerve

Median nerve of Hansen's disease and sequelae are shown in Table 12.39.2.

Table 12.39.1 Ulnar nerve of Hansen's disease and sequelae

	Method of doing	*Finding*	*Significance*
Finger closing pattern	Ask the patient to keep the fingers straight on the table with the palm facing upward. He is then asked to very slowly flex the fingers to bring the tips of the fingers to the palm.	Normally, the MCP joints start moving first and then the IP joints flex to complete the flexion. If the ulnar nerve is involved, the IP joints flex fully and then move the MCP joints.	Denotes paralysis of the primary flexors of the MCP joints. So, the long flexors have to flex the MCP joint and they can do this only after they have fully flexed the IP joints.
Unassisted angle	Ask the patient to make a fist. Then ask him to slowly extend the IP joints alone and bring the IP joints to neutral position, without extending the MCP joints. To make it clear, the surgeon can demonstrate first on his own hand, and then ask the patient to do it on his uninvolved hand if possible.	The patient with ulnar nerve injury will not be able to achieve the lumbrical position. If only the ulnar nerve is involved, the index and middle fingers will come to lumbrical position, but not the ring and little. Now, measure the angle at the PIP joints of the ring and little fingers. This is the unassisted angle.	Denotes paralysis of the primary extensors of the IP joints and flexors of the MCP joints.

Contd...

Contd...

Assisted angle	Now, support the MCP joints of the involved fingers at 90° with your hands and ask the patient to extend the IP joints as above.	The patient may be able to now extend the IP joints and bring them to neutral position. This is because the long extensors of the fingers can extend the IP joints when the MCP joints are stabilized.	If the patient is not able to extend the IP joints fully, it signifies that the long extensors and central slip have become attenuated, most probably due to long standing claw deformity.
Contracture angle	If there is an assisted angle, try to passively extend the proximal interphalangeal (PIP) joints of the involved fingers.	Sometimes, it may not be possible to extend beyond a certain angle. This is the contracture angle.	This signifies that the joint has become stiff due to long standing claw. Hence, it must be corrected either by physiotherapy or surgical means to achieve a full passive range of motion.
Latent clawing	When the patient is asked to keep the involved hand in lumbrical position, he may be able to do it. Test the power of this MCP joint flexion, by giving a short upward push on the volar side of the prophylaxis (PPX) level of the involved fingers.	If the ulnar nerve is involved, the involved fingers will buckle under the pressure and the claw will be revealed.	This signifies that the ulnar nerve is involved, but the soft tissues surrounding the MCP joints are strong enough to stabilize the joint weakly. There is no need to wait for an obvious claw to develop before planning a correction.
Adduction of the fingers	Ask the patient keep all the fingers extended, and insert a card between the fingers. Ask him to grip the card tightly with the sides of his fingers, while the examiner tries to withdraw the card.	In a case of ulnar nerve palsy, the patient will not be able to grip the card properly or not at all.	Indicates paralysis of the adductors of the fingers – the palmar interossei muscles.
Adduction of little finger	Ask the patient to adduct the extended little finger to the extended ring finger.	This will not be possible in a patient with ulnar nerve palsy (Wartenberg's sign).	This is because the third palmar interosseous muscle which must adduct the little finger is paralyzed and only the extensor digiti minimi are acting.
Froment's sign	A book is held by the examiner and the patient is asked to hold it with both hands. The examiner now gently tries to pull the book away, necessitating the patient to apply more pressure with the thumb.	If the ulnar nerve is involved, the involved hand will show increased flexion at the IP joint of the thumb – positive Froment's sign.	If the adductor pollicis muscle, which must act to grip the book is weak, the flexor pollicis longus (FPL) tendon tries to compensate and this manifests as increasing flexion at the IP joint of thumb.

Table 12.39.2 Median nerve of Hansen's disease and sequelae

	Method of doing	*Finding*	*Significance*
Testing for abductor pollicis brevis (APB) muscle	Patient is asked to keep his hand flat on the table, with the palm facing upward. The examiner then holds a pen parallel to the plane of the palm at a distance. He is then asked to lift-up only the thumb to touch the pen. When the patient attempts this, the examiner now palpates the tone of the APB, which is the first palpated muscle on the radial side of the first metacarpal bone.	Sometimes, the patient may be able to weakly touch the pen, only when the level of the pen is brought closer to the palm. Even then, the weakness or absence of muscle tone in APB denotes the involvement of the median nerve.	
Flexor digitorum profundus (FDP) of index and mid	The patient is asked to flex individually only the distal interphalangeal (DIP) joints of the index and middle fingers when the middle phalanx (MPX) segments of the fingers are stabilized by the examiner. When the patient does this, the examiner tests the power of this flexion and at the same time, examines for movement of the DIP joints of the ring and little fingers also.	Patient will not be able to do so individually in a case of high median nerve palsy. There may be some movement of flexion, but this may be by the contiguous movements at the FDP of the ring and little fingers.	Indicates high median nerve palsy.
Testing the FDS action on index finger	The patient is asked to clasp both hands. The position of the index finger is assessed in this position.	When the median nerve is involved at a high level (in the proximal forearm or above), the patient will not be able to flex the IP joints of the index finger and it will remain in extended position (pointing index).	Indicates high median nerve palsy.
Testing the FPL action	Patient is asked to flex the IP joint of the thumb against resistance, while supporting the PPX segment of the thumb.	Will not be possible in high involvement of the median nerve.	Indicates high median nerve palsy.
Thumb web angle	A line is drawn on the dorsal aspect of the hand over the first metacarpal and the second metacarpal bones. The angle between these two lines (the thumb web angle) is measured.	The normal thumb web angle is 40°.	If the angle is less than normal, it indicates tightening of the underlying adductors/stiffness of the carpometacarpal (CMC) joint of thumb and/or the skin. The suppleness of the skin of the thumb web, the free range of movements at CMC joint of thumb must be re-established before planning any tendon transfer.

Contd...

Contd...

Grade of opposition (Kapandji)	The patient is asked to touch the tip of his thumb to the tips of the index, middle, ring and little fingers. The grading of the range of movements is done as shown.	It is important that the patient touches the tips of the fingers with the tip of the thumb. All other pinches are not representative of true opposition.	

Table 12.39.3 **Radial nerve of Hansen's disease and sequelae**

	Method of doing	*Finding*	*Significance*
Extension of fingers	Ask the patient to keep the hand flat on the table with the palm facing downwards. Then, the patient is asked to lift the fingers one by one and each finger is evaluated individually.	The extension of the MCP joints of the fingers is evaluated by this method.	
Extension thumb	The above test is repeated for the thumb, and the patient is asked to actively extend the IP joint of the thumb against resistance.		
Wrist	Patient is asked to make a fist and then extend the wrist against resistance.		

For the Radial Nerve

Radial nerve of Hansen's disease and sequelae are shown in Table 12.39.3.

Position of the joints—should be checked and recorded. This will show any stiffness or contractures and will play an important role in planning the reconstruction. This recording should include both active and passive range of movements. Reversal of the metacarpal arch must also be recorded.

Sensation—the pain, touch sensation should be recorded and the two point discrimination should also be recorded.

Opponensplasty with Flexor Digitorum Superficialis of Ring Finger

40

Introduction

Though there are many procedures for opponensplasty this procedure is a standard one that is commonly used, when the thumb web is tight, and a powerful muscle is needed to overcome this tightness.

Presurgical Counseling

- This procedure is planned to correct only the weak thumb. This surgery will not correct the other problems that may exist on the hand like wasting of the muscles or loss of sensation. These problems need to separate sittings of surgery and cannot usually be combined with the procedure planned at present
- This procedure will be done under axillary block anesthesia
- This procedure will take about 1 hour to perform
- A tendon from the ring finger will be removed and taken to the thumb to make the thumb move in a useful direction. There will be no obvious deficit on the ring finger, but there may be some weakness of the finger
- Admission will be necessary for a minimum period of 3 days
- A dressing will be applied and a plaster of Paris (POP) will be applied, which will be retained for 3 weeks, following which, physiotherapy will be started. This should be continued for a further 3 weeks. During this period of physiotherapy, exercises will be taught to make the tendon of the ring finger move the thumb
- In some instances, the movement that returns on the thumb may be weak and may not be powerful enough for useful work. In some other instances, the tendon may not work at all. This will require another sitting of surgery to correct the problem
- In some instances, the ring finger may develop a minimal deformity on the proximal interphalangeal (PIP) joint. This will require a small surgery to correct the problem
- The general complications of local anesthetic infiltration like hypersensitivity may occur in spite of test dose application. This complication will cause dryness of mouth and apprehension, which can be corrected immediately.

Surgical Steps

1. Prepare the hand as described in Appendix I.
2. Mark the incisions as follows (Fig. 12.40.1):
    - Incision "A"—an incision is marked over the neutral line on the ulnar border of the ring finger about 4 cm long, centered at the level of the PIP joint crease
    - Incision "B"—an incision 2 cm long marked transversely over the distal

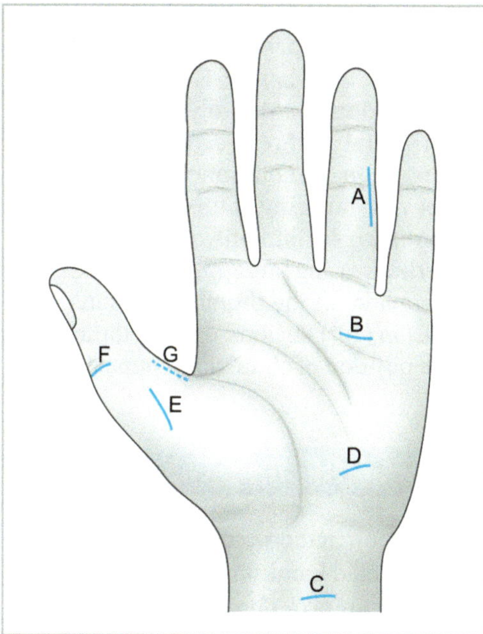

Fig. 12.40.1 Markings for opponensplasty using flexor digitorum superficialis (FDS) of ring finger

palmar crease proximal to the ring finger
- Incision "C"—an incision 2 cm long marked transversely over the flexor aspect of the forearm about 3 cm proximal to the wrist crease
- Incision "D"—an incision 2 cm long marked transversely over the palm just distal and radial to the pisiform bone
- Incision "E"—an incision 2 cm long marked longitudinally over the radial aspect of the thumb at the level of the metacarpophalangeal (MCP) joint just volar to the midpoint
- Incision "F"—an incision 2 cm long marked transversely over the dorsum of the proximal phalanx of the thumb, just proximal to the interphalangeal (IP) joint crease on the thumb.
- Incision "G"—an incision on the ulnar side of the MCP joint of the thumb, about 2 cm long.

3. The tourniquet is raised and the incisions are made.
4. First the incision "A" is made to harvest the FDS tendon. The skin on the volar side is raised superficial to the digital neurovascular bundle. The flexor tendon sheath is identified. An incision is made in the flexor tendon sheath to isolate the flexor digitorum profundus (FDP) and FDS tendons. The FDP tendon is usually seen first and it must be retracted volarward to expose the FDS tendon slips. The ulnar slip is first seen. A hemostat is applied about 1 cm proximal to the insertion. The tendon slip is now cut distal to the hemostat. Now, traction is applied to this cut slip with the hemostat and this will expose the radial slip of the FDS tendon. This slip is also divided 1 cm proximal to the insertion and another hemostat is applied on the proximal cut end. Both hemostats are pulled distally to expose the decussation of the FDS tendon. It is divided with a blade until both slips are free. The vincular attachment will also have to be divided to achieve total release of the FDS slips.
5. Incision "B" is made and the synovium over the FDS and FDP tendons just proximal to the A1 pulley is incised to expose the tendons. Identify the FDS tendon and pull so that the tendon is now delivered in this wound. Suture wound "A" now.
6. The incision "C" is made and the FDS tendon identified among the tendons to the fingers. The FDS of the ring finger is pulled and delivered in the wound.
7. Now, incision "D" is made through the skin and subcutaneous tissues. The subcutaneous fat consisting of fine fat globules is seen. The incision is gently deepened till large fat globules protrude out. Now, a tendon retriever is passed through this wound proximally to exit at the forearm wound. The free end of the FDS tendon is grasped and the tendon delivered at the incision "D".
8. Incision "E" is made through the skin and subcutaneous tissues to expose the insertion of the abductor pollicis brevis tendon. The tendon retriever is passed from this wound to the incision "D". The

free end of the FDS tendon is grasped and retrieved in incision "E". The incisions "B", "C" and "D" are sutured with 4.0 Ethilon.

9. The tendon anchoring is done under correct tension. The wrist is placed in neutral position and the thumb positioned at prone position and abducted position. The thumb should now be facing the middle finger. Now, the free end of the FDS tendon is pulled distally and the excursion of the tendon is recorded. The midpoint of this excursion range is marked and placed close to the tendon of abductor pollicis brevis (APB). It is pulled for 1 cm and the tendon anastomosis is done. The free end of the tendon graft is used to wind around the insertion of the APB tendon and then a suture is applied with 3.0 polypropylenes. The tenodesis effect is checked. When the wrist is flexed, the thumb must open out and when the wrist is flexed, the thumb must oppose to the middle finger.
10. The above method of tendon suturing is done for a case of pure median nerve lesion or injury. If there is a combined median and ulnar nerve injury, the following method of tendon anchorage is done. The anchoring of the tendon is not done only at the APB tendon as discussed above. Two more incisions are made.
11. Incision "F" is made and the extensor pollicis longus (EPL) tendon is identified just proximal to the IP joint.
12. Incision "G" is made and the adductor incision is identified and dissected.
13. At the incision "E", the free end of the FDS tendon is now split into two slips. One slip is passed through a tunnel over the dorsum of the MCP joint of the thumb and attached to the adductor insertion at incision "G" with 4.0 polypropylenes using horizontal mattress suture, under minimal tension as described above. The other slip is passed subcutaneously to incision "F" where it is anchored to the EPL tendon with 4.0 polypropylenes using horizontal mattress suture with neutral tension on the anastomosis.
14. Now, the suturing of the wounds must be done with 4.0 Ethilon.
15. Sterile dressings are applied and a POP slab is applied on the thumb, maintaining the wrist in (10°) flexions, and the thumb kept in a position of abduction - opposition.

Postoperative Protocol

- Admission in the ward
- The affected hand should be kept elevated
- Patient can take normal diet immediately if the procedure was under regional block or after complete recovery if under general anesthesia
- The POP slabs must not be disturbed at all for 3 weeks
- Discharge of the patient by third day
- Patient to retain the POP slab till the end of 3 weeks
- Removal of the POP slab on the 21st day and advise the following:
    - Refer to physiotherapy for active mobilization of the fingers
    - Daily wash with soap and water
    - Massage of scar and grafted skin with coconut oil
    - Patient is advised to continue the mobilization of the fingers; both active and passive and review once every month for evaluation.
    - To continue wearing a short opponens splint at night for 3 weeks after removal of POP.

Opponensplasty with Abductor Digiti Minimi Muscle (Huber's Transfer)

41

Introduction

This method of tendon transfer is ideal for children with weakness of the thenar muscles due to congenital hypoplasia, either of the musculature only, or hypoplasia of the thumb which may occur alone or with hypoplasia of the radius (radial club hand).

Presurgical Counseling

- This procedure is planned to correct only the weak thumb. This surgery will not correct the other problems that may exist on the hand like wasting of the muscles or loss of sensation. These problems need to separate sittings of surgery and cannot usually be combined with the procedure planned at present
- This procedure will be done under axillary block anesthesia
- This procedure will take about 1 hour to perform
- A muscle from the little finger will be removed and taken to the thumb to make the thumb move in a useful direction. There will be no obvious deficit on the little finger, but there may be some weakness of the finger
- Admission will be necessary for a minimum period of 3 days
- A dressing will be applied and a plaster of Paris (POP) will be applied, which will be retained for 3 weeks, following which, physiotherapy will be started. This should be continued for a further 3 weeks. During this period of physiotherapy, exercises will be taught to make the muscle of the little finger move the thumb
- In some instances, the movement that returns on the thumb may be weak and may not be powerful enough for useful work. In some other instances, the muscle may not work at all. This will require another sitting of surgery to correct the problem
- There will be a scar on the palm and the little finger
- The general complications of local anesthetic infiltration like hypersensitivity may occur in spite of test dose application. This complication will cause dryness of mouth and apprehension, which can be corrected immediately.

Surgical Steps

1. Prepare the hand as described in Appendix I.
2. Mark the incisions (Fig. 12.41.1) as follows:
   - First the incision "A" is marked to harvest the abductor digiti minimi (ADM) tendon. First the midpoint on the ulnar neutral line on the proximal phalanx (PPX) segment of the little finger is marked point "P". The point where the neutral line cuts the volar metacarpophalangeal (MCP) joint crease

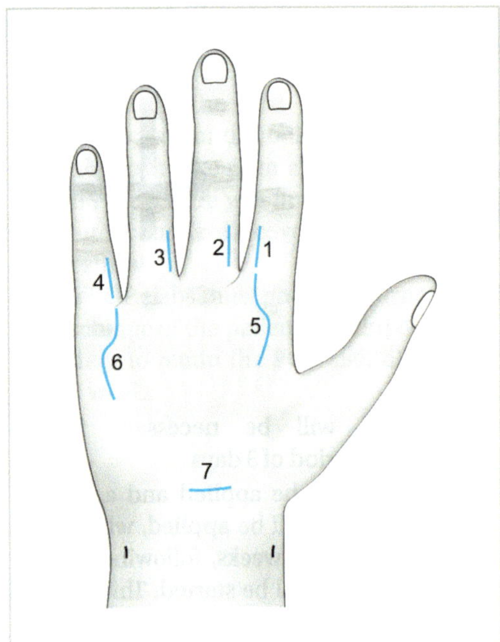

Fig. 12.44.1 Mark the incisions

- Incision "5"—a longitudinally oriented lazy "S" incision over the dorsum of the metacarpophalangeal (MCP) joint of the index finger, extending proximally from incision 1
- Incision "6"—similar to incision 5, but on the dorsal aspect of the MCP joint of the little finger, starting on the radial side of the little finger
- Incision "7"—two centimeter transverse incisions on the dorsum of the hand just distal to the wrist crease, over the base of II MC.

3. The tourniquet is raised and the incisions "1", "2", "3", and "4" are made one by one. The extensor tendon is exposed in the wounds. The portions of the tendon that are exposed are the lateral bands and the central tendon. This can be confirmed by grasping the selected portion of the tendon with a tissue forceps and applying traction proximally. This traction should produce extension of the proximal interphalangeal (PIP) and distal interphalangeal (DIP) joints. This must be done on all the fingers. A moist gauze piece is placed over the incisions.
4. The incision "5" is now made through skin, down through the subcutaneous tissues to the extensor tendons. The extensor indicis proprius (EIP) tendon is identified. This is the more ulnar of the two extensor tendons to the index finger. The two extensor tendons together form the extensor expansion. Surgeons require a good length of the EIP tendon. Hence, harvesting the tendon alone is not enough, and an extension will have to be taken from the extensor expansion. This is done with a number 15 blade and about 3 cm length is taken beyond the MCP joint level. Now, a hemostat is applied over the free end of the EIP tendon, and a saline gauze is placed over the tendon.
5. The incision "6" is made similar to incision "5", but over the little finger. The extensor digiti minimi (EDM) tendon is harvested just as the EIP was harvested. The EDM tendon is the more ulnar tendon of the two extensor tendons to the little finger. A hemostat is applied over the free end of the EDM tendon.
6. Now, incision "7" is made, after confirming the position of the marking by applying traction on the hemostats holding the free ends of the EIP and EDM tendons, and palpating the movement of the tendons beneath the skin of the marking. The EIP and EDM tendons are identified and isolated. They are pulled and this maneuver delivers the two tendons at incision "7".
7. Each tendon is divided longitudinally into two slips. This is done by holding the two corners of the free ends with hemostats and using a number 11 blade to split the tendon. Remember to keep bathing the tendon with normal saline while doing this. Thus, there are now four tendon slips; two from splitting the EIP and two from the EDM. The radial and ulnar slips

from the EIP tendon will be used for the index and middle fingers respectively. The radial and ulnar slips from the EDM tendon will be used for the ring and little fingers respectively. The splitting should stop proximally at the site of incision "7". Now, incisions "5" and "6" can be closed with 4.0 Ethilon.

8. Flex the MCP joint of the index finger to 90° and pass the tendon retriever through incision "1" to exit at incision "7". While doing this, the retriever must be advanced very gently, making probing maneuvers to find the path of least resistance. The retriever must not be forced into any path. It must be remembered that this route must be volar to the deep transverse metacarpal ligament. Grasp the radial most slip of the four tendon slips and pull it gently to deliver it in incision "1". Similarly, the other slips must be delivered into the respective incisions "2", "3" and "4". Suture incision "8".
9. The distal tendon anastomosis is done now, by suturing the free end of the tendon slip to the portion of the extensor tendon that has already been dissected and kept ready. While suturing, it is important to adjust the tension correctly.
10. First, the index finger is dealt with. The hand is placed in a position with rolled up towels of 30° flexion at wrist, 60° flexion at MCP joints of all fingers and fingers straight. Now, the free end of the fascia lata graft slip is pulled gently at the incision "1" and the movement of the tendon is assessed. Usually, there will be about 2 cm of excursion. Suture the midpoint of this excursion to the portion of the extensor tendon that has already been dissected and kept ready. Check whether this suturing is too tight or lose by the tenodesis effect and adjust the tension as necessary.
11. Next, repeat the procedure for the little finger, suturing the tendons at a point just distal to the midpoint of the excursion of the tendon slip of EDM. This is to provide slightly more traction on the little finger to correct the metacarpal arch reversal to a certain extent.
12. Now, the suturing must be done on the middle and ring fingers. The ulnar slip of the divided EIP tendon is used for the middle finger and the radial slip of the divided EDM is used for the ring finger. Then all the incisions "1", "2", "3" and "4" must be closed with 4.0 Ethilon, and the tourniquet released.
13. Sterile dressings are applied and two POP slabs are applied, one on the volar aspect and another on the dorsal aspect. The position of the hand to be maintained is wrist in neutral position, MCP joints of fingers in 90° flexion and interphalangeal (IP) joints of the fingers straight.

Postoperative Protocol

- Admission in the ward
- The affected hand should be kept elevated
- Patient can take normal diet immediately if the procedure was under regional block or after complete recovery if under general anesthesia
- The POP slabs must not be disturbed at all
- Discharge of the patient by third day
- Patient to retain the POP slab till the end of 3 weeks
- Removal of the POP slab on the 21st day and advise the following:
  - Refer to physiotherapy for active mobilization of the fingers
  - Daily wash with soap and water
  - Massage of scar and grafted skin with coconut oil
  - Patient is advised to continue the mobilization of the fingers; both active and passive and review once every month for evaluation.

tendon end reaches. The free end of the PT tendon is pulled maximally and then released. The amount of excursion of the tendon is noted. The midpoint of this excursion range is noted. The PT tendon is now slightly pulled and the tendon anastomosis is now done. The technique of tendon anastomosis is as follows:

- The tendon anastomosis is done by Pulvertaft weave. Hold the ECRB tendon taut with a hemostat applied on the end and pulling proximally
- About 1 cm proximal to the end of the tendon, make a cut in a volar to dorsal direction with a number 11 blade, with just enough length to allow the PT tendon end through. Pull the tendon end through. Apply a suture with 3.0 polypropylene using horizontal mattress sutures
- About 1 cm proximal to the first cut, make another cut with number 11 blade, from a radial to ulnar direction. Thread the free end of the PT tendon end through this opening also and suture with 3.0 polypropylene using horizontal mattress sutures.

8. When the tendon anastomosis is over, the extra length of the PT tendon is trimmed.
9. It must be made that the wrist can be passively flexed and the tendon anastomosis is not too tight as to prevent it.
10. Now, incision "C" is made and the palmaris longus (PL) tendon is dissected at this level by freeing it from the numerous fibrous strands that connect it to the overlying skin and the surrounding structures. Once it is totally dissected, it is divided and a hemostat applied on the cut end.
11. Incision "D" is made after applying traction on the cut end of the tendon and palpating the taut tendon under the skin. The tendon is dissected in this wound.
12. The PL is retrieved through this wound, and the hemostat reapplied at the cut end. Moist gauze is placed over the length of the tendon lying outside.
13. Incision "F" is made. Care must be taken to avoid injury to the radial artery and the superficial branch of the radial nerve at this area. A tendon retriever is passed from this incision, proximally to the incision "D", the end of the PL is grasped and pulled to be delivered in incision "F". Moist gauze is placed around the free end of the tendon.
14. Now, in incision "B", the EPL tendon is identified as proximal as possible. This tendon lies in the third compartment and can be identified by the extension produced on the thumb interphalangeal (IP) joint by traction proximally. The tendon is divided.
15. Now, incision "E" is made. The EPL tendon is identified on the dorsal aspect of the thumb and dissected from the extensor pollicis brevis (EPB) tendon which lies to the radial side. Now, traction is applied and the EPL tendon is delivered into the incision "E". The exposed length of the tendon is covered with saline gauze.
16. From incision "F", a tendon retriever is passed through to incision "E" and the free end of the EPL tendon is grasped and pulled to be delivered in incision "F" itself. The incision "E" is closed primarily with 4.0 Ethilon.
17. The tendon anastomosis between the PL and the EPL tendon is done now in the site of incision "F". The tendon anastomosis is done by the Pulveraft weave as described above. The PL tendon's free end is woven into the proximal end of the EPL tendon after adjusting the tension. With the wrist maintained at 45° extensions, a trial stitch is made between the ends of the PL and the EPL. When the wrist is gently passively flexed, the thumb must extend.
18. Now, the incision "C" is explored again and the tendon of flexor carpi radialis (FCR) is identified. This tendon is radial to the PL tendon that has already been divided. Now, the FCR tendon is divided as distally as possible.

19. Through the incision "D", the FCR tendon is identified and pulled so that the free end is delivered in incision "D" itself.
20. In incision "B", the tendons of the extensor digitorum are identified and dissected. This includes the extensor digitorum communis (EDC) to index, middle, ring, little, the extensor indicis proprius (EIP) tendon and the extensor digiti minimi (EDM) tendon. A tendon retriever is passed from this wound to the incision "D" around the radial border of the forearm and the free end of the FCR tendon is grasped and delivered into incision "B".
21. Now, the tourniquet is released and hemostasis achieved. Except incision "B", all the other wounds are closed primarily with 4.0 Ethilon.
22. Now, the tension adjustment is done. Each tendon of the extensor to the finger is pulled to note the movement. The tendon is now pulled enough to hold the finger in a position of extension at the MCP joints (not hyperextension). The free end of FCR tendon is now woven through the extensors of the fingers after making a longitudinal cut in the extensor tendons in a radio ulnar direction with number 11 blade. Before making the cut in the extensor tendon, the position of the fingers is ascertained. After the FCR passes through each tendon, an anchoring stitch is made with 3.0 polypropylene. In this way all the tendons are woven to the FCR tendon. Now, the tenodesis effect is checked. On wrist flexion, there must be hyperextension of the MCP joints of the fingers.
23. Incision "B" is closed primarily with 4.0 Ethilon.
24. Sterile dressings are applied and a volar POP slab is applied, keeping the wrist in 45° extension, the finger MCP joints in 30° flexion and the IP joints of the fingers straight. Another POP slab is applied on the volar aspect of the thumb, holding it in palmar abduction at the carpometacarpal (CMC) joint, and extension at the MCP and IP joints.

Postoperative Protocol

- Admission in the ward
- The affected hand should be kept elevated
- Patient can take normal diet immediately if the procedure was under regional block or after complete recovery if under general anesthesia
- The POP slabs must not be disturbed at all
- Discharge of the patient by third day
- Patient to retain the POP slab till the end of 3 weeks
- Removal of the POP slab on the 21st day and advise the following:
    - Refer to physiotherapy for active mobilization of the fingers
    - Daily wash with soap and water
    - Massage of scar and grafted skin with coconut oil
    - Patient is advised to continue the mobilization of the fingers; both active and passive and review once every month for evaluation.

SECTION

13

Congenital Disorders

Congenital Disorders—Assessment

46

Introduction

Dealing with the classification, assessment and the surgical management of all the congenital anomalies is beyond the scope of this manual. However, the most common conditions will be dealt here, so that the beginner will be able to do the basic surgical procedures. As it has been stressed earlier, reading this manual will not be enough knowledge to perform the surgery straightaway. A thorough study of the classification, nomenclature and altered anatomy are essential before surgery can be attempted.

The following chapters will deal with six different congenital anomalies seen commonly:

- Syndactyly
- Radial club hand
- Trigger finger and trigger thumb
- Macrodactyly
- Polydactyly
- Cleft hand.

Congenital anomalies as a whole have some features that should be assessed. In addition, each condition has peculiar assessment criteria, which are also mentioned here.

Assessment Criteria—General

The Details that Must be Collected are:

- *Consanguinity:* This is particularly relevant in our country where marriage between uncles and nieces and between first cousins is allowed, and sometimes even encouraged.
- *Antenatal history:* Any relevant antenatal history must be obtained like history of exanthematous fevers, ingestion of drugs, exposure to radiation and smoking. The outbreak of phocomelia, a severe congenital deformity occurring in the babies born of mothers who had taken the drug thalidomide, is well known.
- *Family history:* Congenital anomalies like syndactyly are known to occur in families.

Assessment Criteria—Specific

These will be dealt with under the specific conditions.

Syndactyly

47

Assessment (Syndactyly)

- *Fingers involved:* Commonly involves the middle and ring fingers, but any of the fingers and any number of fingers may be involved. This is important especially in planning the management protocol.
- Whether both upper limbs are involved
- Whether the lower limbs are involved
  - *Any other congenital anomalies:* The type of syndactyly will be typical if it is a part of a congenital syndrome. For example, in apert syndrome, all the fingers are involved in the syndactyly forming a spade like hand, and typically involve both upper limbs. There are also many features suggestive of the particular syndrome.
- *Type of the syndactyly (length):*
  - If the entire length of the fingers is involved, it denotes complete syndactyly.
  - If only part of the length of the finger is involved, it denotes incomplete syndactyly.
- *Type of syndactyly (involvement of bones):*
  - If there is no fusion of the skeletal components between the syndactylized fingers, it is referred to as simple syndactyly.
  - If there is a fusion of even a part of the skeleton of the fingers, it is referred to as complex syndactyly.
- *Special types of syndactyly:*
  - *Acrosyndactyly:* This is a slightly different condition, even though the fingers are in syndactyly. The pathogenesis of this condition is different, in that, the fingers have usually developed normally, but due to some intrauterine problem, parts of the fingers have got amputated and have healed *in utero*.
    - Typically, there will be gaps between the syndactylized fingers that run through from the palmar to the dorsal side.
    - There will be irregular tips of the fingers.
  - *Apert syndrome:* The syndactyly of the hand in this condition has been described above.

Management Schedule

Factors to be considered while planning the treatment:

- *Age of the child:* There is no specific age limit for surgery on syndactyly. It can be done as early as 6 months also. It is also important that the surgery should not be delayed beyond 4 years, when the child enters school. So, it must be planned in such a way that all surgery is over for the hand by the age of 4 years.
- *Bilateral involvement:* If both hands are involved, both can be operated on at the same time; especially if two operating teams are available. This is to minimize the period of anesthesia and to reduce the number of surgical stages. However, if the patient is an adult (which is sometimes

possible), it is ideal that bilateral syndactyly is operated on in two stages, because it will avoid making the patient totally dependent on others following plaster of Paris (POP) slabs on both hands.

- *Fingers involved:* If the thumb or little fingers are involved, they must be released first. If the index finger and ring finger are involved together with the middle finger, the index finger must be released first. So, the priority of importance of the fingers release is as follows:
  - Thumb
  - Little finger
  - Index finger
  - Middle finger
  - Ring finger.

Principles of planning for syndactyly surgery:

- If the thumb, little or index fingers are involved, surgery must be done as early as possible after 6 months age.
- Do not operate on adjacent sides of a finger at the same time. For example, if there is a syndactyly between the index, middle and ring finger, do not release all the fingers at the same time. Only one can be released, either the index and middle or the ring and middle fingers. According to principle A, the index and middle fingers should be released first.
- The timing between two stages must be a minimum of 6 months.

Surgery (Syndactyly)

Presurgical Counseling

- The surgery will be done under general anesthesia. Both hands will be operated on at the same time (in children).
- A POP slab will be applied from the elbow to the fingers after the surgery on the operated upper limb.
- If necessary, a skin graft will be harvested from the groin region. There will be a small scar on the groin region, but there will be no other deficit.
- Admission will be necessary for a minimum of 3 days.
- The child can take fluids 4 hours after the surgery.
- There may be minimal pain in the first post-operative night. Analgesics and sedatives may be necessary.
- The POP will be removed after 2 weeks. A short anesthesia may be required when this is done, if the child is too small to cooperate.
- After the POP is removed, splints will be required for as long as the surgeon feels necessary.
- In some instances, there may be small problems, like creeping forward of the web, contracture of the finger. This will need surgical correction at a later date.

Surgical Steps

1. After the anesthesia is administered and patient put in supine position, the hand is prepared as described in Appendix I.
2. The markings are now made (Figs 13.47.1A and B):
   - The fingers are flexed at the meta-carpophalangeal (MCP) joints and the knuckles of the two fingers are marked. Similarly, the dorsum of the proximal interphalangeal (PIP) joints is also marked with a single point in the midline.
   - The midline of the dorsum and the midline of the volar aspect of the fingers are marked.
   - With the markings on the MCP joints as base, the dorsal flap "D" is marked. The length of this flap should be two-thirds of the distance between the MCP joint and the PIP joint. This flap should have a lesser length on the side of the "important finger" (between the middle and ring, it is the ring finger; between the middle and index, it is the index finger). Thus, the advancing edge of the dorsal flap will be sloping.
   - The palmar rectangular flap will be marked now. Expose the palm of the

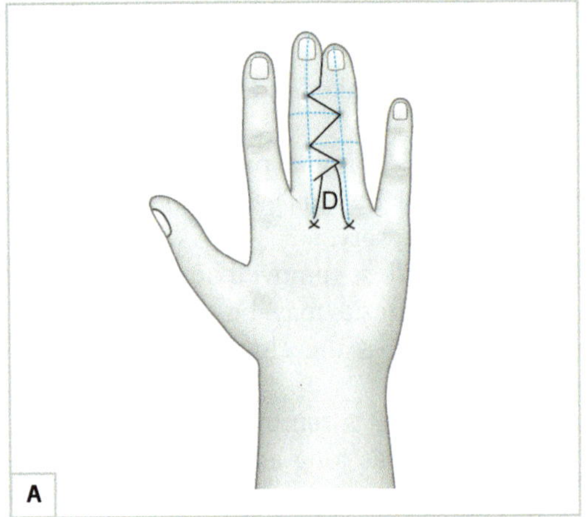

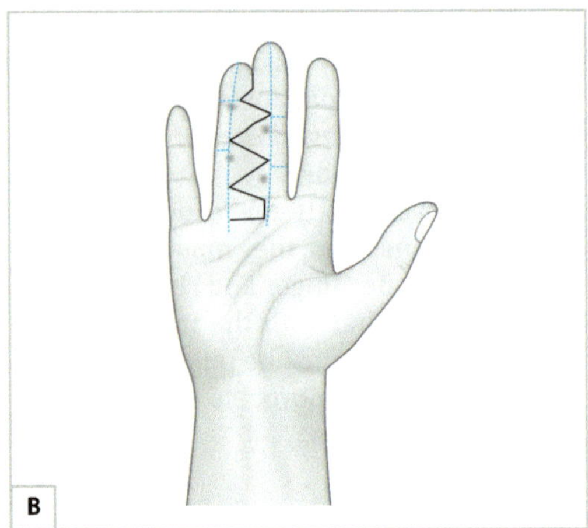

Figs 13.47.1A and B Markings for syndactyly release

hand. Flex the fingers at the MCP joints of the involved fingers. There will be a flexion crease at a particular point. This is the level of the proximal limb of the rectangular flap. The rectangular flap should be based on the "important finger". The length of the flap should be the width of the dorsal flap "D".

- Now, the dorsal zig-zag incisions can be marked on the fingers. The first dorsal triangular flap is marked based on the "nonimportant finger". The flaps should not cross the marked midline on the dorsum or on the volar aspect of the fingers. Beyond the distal interphalangeal (DIP) joints, the incision becomes straight and ends on the tip of the finger.
- Draw dotted lines from the tips of the dorsal flaps backward over the middle of the flap in a horizontal line to the point on the volar midline. This is the point where the tip of the dorsal flap will reach. At this point, it should be the apex of the palmar triangular flaps.
- The first palmar triangular flap is based on the "important finger". All the palmar triangular flaps are then drawn as dictated by the dotted lines.

3. Now, the tourniquet can be raised.
4. The incisions are made in the following order. First the dorsal flap is raised. This is raised after making the incisions up to the skin and subcutaneous tissues and raising the flap with a layer of subcutaneous fat. The other dorsal incisions are made and the respective dorsal triangular flaps raised in the same plane.
5. Now, the palmar aspect is exposed and the rectangular flap is raised first. The other palmar triangular flaps are raised.
6. Now, the soft tissues between the two fingers are dissected. The digital neurovascular bundle is identified. There are usually two bundles, one for each finger. Occasionally, there may be only one bundle. This can be allocated for one of the fingers and the two fingers now divided. The proximal extent of the division between the fingers is determined by the point of division of the proper digital artery. If the division of the digital nerve is very distal, it can be separated by gently teasing the epineurium between the two digital branches. The viability of the fingers is ascertained before proceeding to the next step.
7. The soft tissues can be defatted by excising the fat globules, while carefully preserving

the neurovascular bundles. This step helps to reduce the bulk on the finger and thus ensures a tensionless suturing of the flaps and avoids complications in the postoperative period.

8. Moist saline gauze is placed over the entire length of the wound and gentle compression applied. The hand is elevated and the tourniquet released. After 3 minutes, the hand is kept back on the table and hemostasis achieved.
9. The suturing of the flaps is now done. First the dorsal rectangular flap "D" is sutured to the volar aspect to create the commissure. Next the palmar rectangular flap is brought round the side of the finger and sutured to the skin edge on the dorsum. All the dorsal and palmar triangular flaps are thus sutured using 4.0 vicryl. There will be one or two small areas without skin cover. A full thickness skin graft should be harvested from the lateral end of the groin crease and applied over the raw areas. Anchoring of the skin graft is done with 4.0 vicryl.
10. The hand and fingers are cleaned thoroughly and nonadherent dressings applied. Fluffy gauze pieces are applied between the fingers and sterile dressings applied. An above elbow POP slab is applied.

Postoperative Protocol

- Admission in the ward.
- The affected hand should be kept elevated.
- Patient can take normal diet after complete recovery if under general anesthesia.
- Discharge of the patient by third day.
- Inspection of the suture line after 10 days only. If necessary, a short general anesthesia may be required if the child is very anxious. Suture removal can be done on the same day. The POP slab can also be removed. The following are advised:
  - Refer to physiotherapy for active mobilization of the fingers
  - Daily wash with soap and water
  - Massage of scar and grafted skin with coconut oil
  - Patient is advised to continue the mobilization of the fingers; both active and passive and review once every month for evaluation.

Cleft Hand

48

Assessment (Cleft Hand)

In addition to the general assessment criteria outlined in the earlier chapter, there are certain criteria to be assessed specifically in a cleft hand. The first assessment is to analyze the type of cleft.

Typical Cleft

There is no middle finger ray. So, the index and thumb fingers stay on the radial side and the ring and little fingers are on the ulnar side.

Atypical Cleft

There is absence of more than one ray.

There are certain characteristics to help and differentiate between the two types of cleft (Table 13.48.1).

Features to look for that indicate the severity of the problem:

- Deficiency of middle finger ray
- Web contracture between the thumb and index fingers
- Syndactyly between the ring and little fingers
- Sometimes defect of middle finger ray
- Sometimes defect of index finger ray
- Sometimes even the thumb is absent.

There are certain bony deformities that may be seen:

- Loss of one metacarpal—usual
- Bifid metacarpal—supporting two fingers
- Two metacarpals—supporting one finger
- Sometimes transverse orientation of metacarpal is seen.

Table 13.48.1 Characteristics to help and differentiate between typical cleft and atypical cleft

Typical cleft	*Atypical cleft*
"V"-shaped defect	"U"-shaped defect
Bilateral	Unilateral
Involves feet	Does not involve feet
Inherited	Sporadic

Functional Problems

There are usually not many functional problems; this condition is more of a cosmetic problem. Surgery may be indicated only in certain situations.

Management Protocol

Management protocol of cleft hand is shown in Table 13.48.2.

Simple Closure of the Cleft—Method of Barsky

Presurgical Counseling

- The surgery will be done under general anesthesia. Both hands can be operated on at the same time (in children).

Table 13.48.2 Management protocol of cleft hand

Finding	*Surgery indicated*	*Method*
Typical cleft	Simple closure of the cleft	Barsky method
Thumb web contracture	Release of contracture and closure of cleft	Littler method
Syndactyly between ring and little	Syndactyly release	Discussed in earlier chapter
Bony deformities	Relevant osteotomies	

- A plaster of Paris (POP) slab will be applied from the elbow to the fingers after the surgery on the operated upper limb.
- This surgery is only to bring the two deviated fingers together. If there are already some other deformities like contracture of fingers or syndactyly of fingers, they will be dealt with at a different stage.
- Admission will be necessary for a minimum of 3 days.
- The child can take fluids 4 hours after the surgery.
- There may be minimal pain in the first postoperative night. Analgesics and sedatives may be necessary.
- The POP will be removed after 2 weeks. A short anesthesia may be required when this is done, if the child is too small to cooperate.
- After the POP is removed, splints will be required for as long as the surgeon feels necessary.
- In some instances, there may be small problems, like creeping forward of the web, contracture of the finger. This will need surgical correction at a later date.

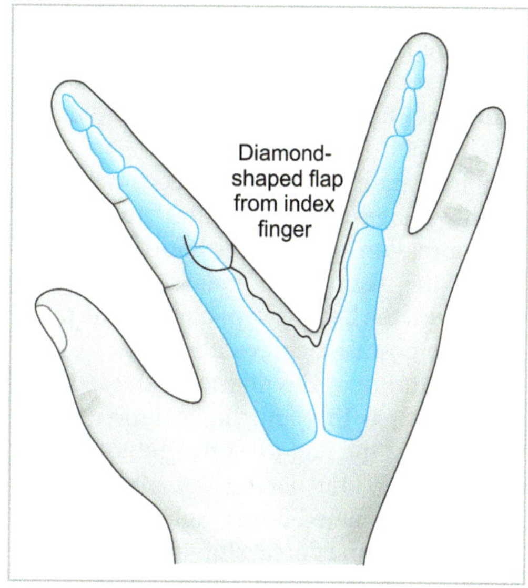

Fig. 13.48.1 Markings for the flap

Surgical Steps

- The hand is first prepared as described in Appendix I.
- The markings are made now (Fig. 13.48.1).
    - The commissural flap is first marked. This flap is diamond shaped and distally based on the proximal phalanx region of one of the fingers. The base of the flap AB is designed at the level of the junction between the proximal and distal half of the proximal phalanx. The dorsal midline and the volar midline axes are marked. The flap is marked from mid-dorsal line to mid-volar line. The length of the flap is equal to its width. The base is marked in such a way that the volar point of the base "B" is more distal than the dorsal point "A".
    - On the opposing finger, a transverse line FG is marked at the junction of proximal and distal half.
    - The incision is marked on the cleft region.
- The tourniquet is raised up to 200 mm Hg and the incisions are made down through the skin and subcutaneous tissues. The diamond-shaped flap is raised.

- Any remnants of abnormal bone, either bifid metacarpal, or double metacarpal or transversely-oriented bone should be dealt with now.
- Soft tissues are dissected around the neck of the two metacarpals on either side of the cleft. They are sutured together using nonabsorbable suture material—3.0 polypropylene. This is done to replace the transverse metacarpal ligament and bring the two fingers together. Sometimes, if the second metacarpal bone does not yield, it may be necessary to do an osteotomy on the base of the second metacarpal to allow the index finger to get approximated to the ring finger.
- Moist saline gauze is placed over the entire length of the wound and gentle compression applied. The hand is elevated and the tourniquet released. After 3 minutes, the hand is kept back on the table and hemostasis achieved.
- The suturing of the diamond-shaped flap is done first. This suturing is done in such a way that the flap does not get anchored transversely, but facing dorsally, so that the newly created finger web has a gentle normal looking dorsal slope (Fig. 13.48.2).
- Suturing is done with 4.0 polyamide sutures. Drainage tubes are kept at strategic positions.
- The hand and fingers are cleaned thoroughly and nonadherent dressings applied. Fluffy gauze pieces are applied between the fingers and sterile dressings applied. An above elbow POP slab is applied with the elbow in 90° flexion and the forearm kept in mid-prone position.

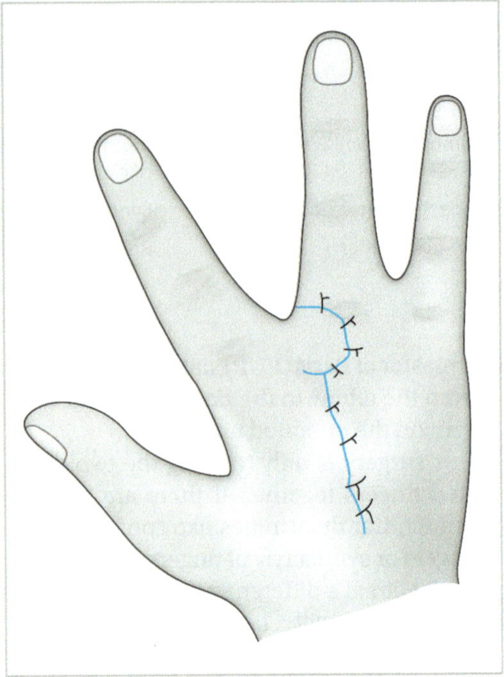

Fig. 13.48.2 Final suturing

Postoperative Protocol

- Admission in the ward.
- The affected hand should be kept elevated.
- Patient can take normal diet after complete recovery if under general anesthesia.
- Discharge of the patient by third day.
- Inspection of the suture line after 10 days only. If necessary, a short general anesthesia may be required if the child is very anxious. Suture removal can be done on the same day. The POP slab needs to be retained for another 2 weeks.
- After a further 2 weeks, the POP is removed. *The following are advised:*
  - Refer to physiotherapy for active mobilization of the fingers
  - Daily wash with soap and water
  - Massage of scar and grafted skin with coconut oil
  - A splint must be applied to maintain the index and ring fingers in approximated position and a static thumb web spacer must be incorporated in the splint. This splint must be maintained for a minimum of a further 3 weeks.
- Child is encouraged to continue the mobilization of the fingers; both active and passive and review once every month for evaluation.

Release of Adduction Contracture of Thumb and Closure of the Cleft (Method of Littler)

Presurgical Counseling

- The surgery will be done under general anesthesia. Both hands can be operated on at the same time (in children).
- This surgery is only to separate the thumb and index fingers and also to bring the two deviated fingers together. Hence, this surgery is mainly for the cosmetic correction of the deformity. There is some chance that the already present function may be compromised to some extent in the beginning due to the scars of surgery. If there are already some other deformities like contracture of fingers or syndactyly of fingers, they will be dealt with at a different stage.
- There may be need for skin grafting to cover some raw areas. If so, the graft will be harvested from the thigh, and a dressing applied over this area, which will heal spontaneously in a period of about 2 weeks. Sometimes, if the requirement of graft is small, the graft will be taken from the groin crease, and in this situation, the wound will be closed leading to a scar that will settle in the groin crease line.
- A POP slab will be applied from the elbow to the fingers after the surgery on the operated upper limb.
- The child can take fluids 4 hours after the surgery.
- There may be minimal pain in the first postoperative night. Analgesics and sedatives may be necessary.
- Admission will be necessary for a minimum of 3 days.
- The POP will be removed after 2 weeks. A short anesthesia may be required when this is done, if the child is too small to cooperate.
- After the POP is removed, splints will be required for as long as the surgeon feels necessary.
- In some instances, there may be small problems, like creeping forward of the web, contracture of the finger. This will need surgical correction at a later date.

Surgical Steps

- This surgery is usually done under general anesthesia.
- The hand is first prepared as described in Appendix I.
- The markings are made now (Figs 13.48.3A and B).
- Mark the mid-dorsal line, neutral line and the mid-volar line on the index finger and the ring fingers. The neutral line will travel on the margins of the cleft. Now, mark a point at the junction of the proximal third and middle third of the proximal phalanx region on the neutral line on the ulnar side of the index finger (A) and the radial side of the ring finger (B). Mark another point "C" about 1 cm proximal to the edge of the cleft on the dorsum of the hand.
- Join the points AC and BC, running between the mid-dorsal line and the neutral lines of the corresponding fingers.
- At the point A, make a longitudinal incision distally along the neutral line up to the middle of the proximal phalanx. Similarly on the ring finger, mark a distally based flap YBZ of sides measuring equal to the distance AX.
- On the volar aspect, mark a line from the point "A" that travels in between the mid-volar line and the neutral line of the index finger up to a point "D" that does not extend beyond the volar apex of the cleft. Similarly draw another line from the point "B" that travels between the mid-volar line of the ring finger and its neutral line to a point "E" that extends slightly beyond the volar apex of the cleft.

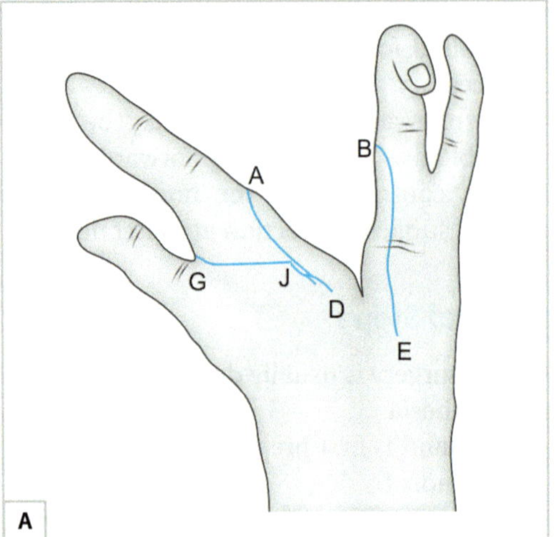

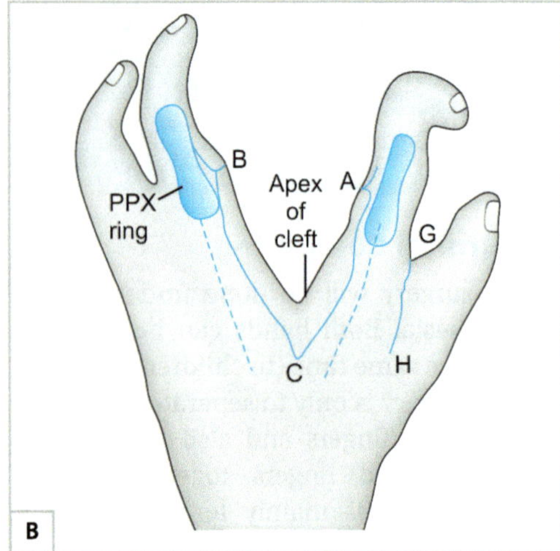

Figs 13.48.3A and B Marking of the incisions

> The blood supply of this flap is from the skin bridge formed by DE. Hence, it is safer to make the lines AD and BE diverging slightly rather than run strictly parallel.

- Now, a marking is made to release the thumb web. Mark the point "G" where the index finger and the thumb meet at the web. From this point, a line is marked extending proximally on the dorsal aspect of the hand up to the point "H" at the junction between the bases of the first and second metacarpal bones. Now, a marking is made on the volar aspect from the point "G" to a point "J" on the midpoint of the already marked line AD. This creates a triangular flap of skin on the volar aspect of the index finger.
- The tourniquet is raised up to 200 mm Hg and the incisions are made down through the skin and subcutaneous tissues in the space between the index and ring fingers. The flap is raised carefully, taking care to avoid injury to the neurovascular bundles of the index and ring fingers. In this way, the flap DCE is based only on the volar skin and soft tissues and this flap of skin is being planned to resurface thumb web that is going to be created. Sometimes the third metacarpal bone may be present, either fully, or as a stump. It is ideal to remove the metacarpal at the base, so that the index metacarpal can be transposed onto this stump while reconstructing the finger. Any remnants of abnormal bone, either bifid metacarpal or double metacarpal or transversely oriented bone is also dealt with now.
- Now, the incisions GH and GJ are made through skin and subcutaneous tissues. As the incision is deepened, care must be taken to avoid injury to the neurovascular bundles on the thumb and index fingers. The adductor pollicis muscle comes into view on the volar side of the wound now. This must be erased from the second metacarpal to get a good release. The first dorsal interosseous muscle also must be divided near the base of the first metacarpal. Care must be taken at this dissection to avoid injuring the radial artery that passes between the two heads of the adductors. These steps alone may not achieve a good thumb web, as the index metacarpal may still be tilted toward the thumb.
- At this point, the index finger is held only by the metacarpal, long flexors and extensors and neurovascular bundles. The base of the

second metacarpal can be osteotomized to free the index finger, so that it can be moved radially over the stump of the third metacarpal bone. It can be fixed at its new position with short K-wires.

- When the finger is shifted in this way, there is a high chance that it scissors with the ring finger. Hence, it is necessary while fixing the second metacarpal, to rotate it slightly to face the volar aspect.
- This alone may not be necessary to retain the position of the index finger in alignment with the ring finger. Soft tissues are dissected around the neck of the two metacarpals on either side of the cleft. They are sutured together using nonabsorbable suture material—3.0 polypropylene. This is done to replace the transverse metacarpal ligament and bring the two fingers together.
- The flap DCE is now transposed to the newly created thumb web. Moist saline gauze is placed over the entire length of the wound and gentle compression applied. The hand is elevated and the tourniquet released. After 3 minutes, the hand is kept back on the table and hemostasis achieved.
- The flap DCE is now sutured with 4.0 polyamide suture. This flap may not be adequate to cover the entire raw area in the thumb web, but it is important to resurface the raw area adjacent to the thumb to ensure that the web does not undergo any contracture. The raw area if any on the radial side of the index finger side can be covered with a full thickness graft from the groin, or a thick split thickness graft from the thigh.
- The wound is now sutured with 4.0 polyamide on the space between the index finger and the ring finger (Figs 13.48.4A and B). The commissural flap YBZ is sutured to the defect created by the incision AX, to form a healthy finger commissure.
- Drainage tubes are kept at strategic positions.
- The hand and fingers are cleaned thoroughly and nonadherent dressings applied. Fluffy gauze pieces are applied between the fingers and sterile dressings applied. An above elbow POP slab is applied with the elbow in 90° flexion and the forearm kept in mid-prone position.

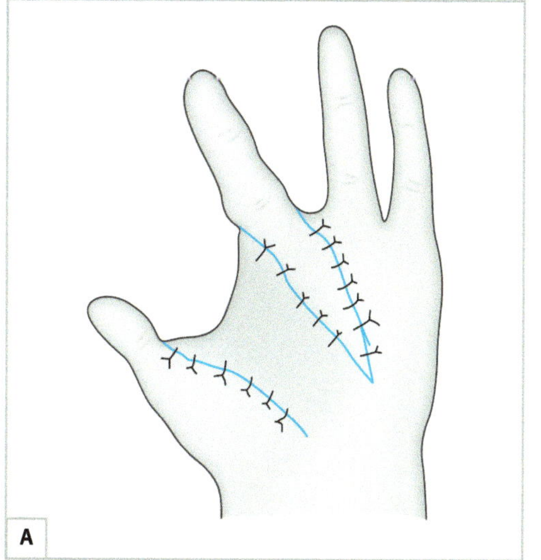

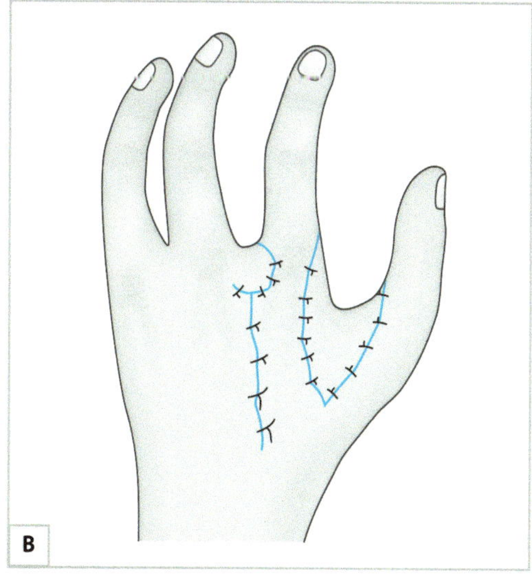

Figs 13.48.4A and B Suturing of the skin flaps

Postoperative Protocol

- Admission in the ward.
- The affected hand should be kept elevated.
- Patient can take normal diet after complete recovery if under general anesthesia.
- Discharge of the patient by third day.
- Inspection of the suture line after 10 days only. If necessary, a short general anesthesia may be required if the child is very anxious. Suture removal can be done on the same day. The POP slab needs to be retained for another 2 weeks.
- After a further 2 weeks, the POP is removed. *The following are advised:*
- Refer to physiotherapy for active mobilization of the fingers
- Daily wash with soap and water
- Massage of scar and grafted skin with coconut oil
- A splint must be applied to maintain the index and ring fingers in approximated position and a static thumb web spacer must be incorporated in the splint. This splint must be maintained for a minimum of a further 3 weeks.
- Child is encouraged to continue the mobilization of the fingers; both active and passive and review once every month for evaluation.

Trigger Thumb Release

49

Introduction

One of the most common congenital conditions affecting the hand is the congenital trigger thumb. This may be commonly a bilateral condition. The treatment of this affliction consists of surgical release. The release of this trigger thumb should be done as early as possible to preserve the function of the thumb.

Surgical Steps

- Bilateral release of the trigger thumb can be done simultaneously. The preferred anesthesia is general anesthesia, or sedation with infiltration of local anesthetic solution. The combination of local anesthesia and sedation is preferred, but done when the patient is a little older and can cooperate for the procedure.
- The affected hand is painted and prepared as in Appendix I. If surgery is planned on both hands, both hands are prepared and draped and kept ready.
- The tourniquet is raised up to 200 mm Hg.
- The volar aspect of the thumb is palpated. There will be a nodular swelling at the level of the metacarpophalangeal (MCP) joint. A transverse incision is marked at the level of the volar MCP crease of the thumb, measuring about 1.0 cm in length. The incision need not go from one neutral line to the other.
- Make the incision on the marking with a No. 15 blade. The incision must be made very gently and should be superficial. This is because the digital nerves are very superficial in this condition and may be injured by an inadvertent deep incision. Once the incision goes through the skin to the underlying fat, skin hooks are applied to both edges and the skin edges lifted up.
- Dissection is now done in a longitudinal direction on either side of the flexor tendon sheath which runs in the mid-volar line. This dissection aims at mobilizing both neurovascular bundles the lie on both sides of the flexor tendon sheath and run parallel to it. Once they are dissected, they can be retracted to either side, so that they can be prevented from getting injured during the surgery on the tendon sheath.
- Now, the tendon sheath has been dissected free from the neurovascular bundles. Palpate the sheath and find the nodular swelling at the level of the A1 pulley.
- Make an incision with a No. 15 blade on one side of the tendon sheath. This incision must also be made carefully as the tendon of flexor pollicis longus (FPL) lies immediately below the sheath and should not be injured. The incision must be extended both proximally and distally as far as possible. When this incision is completed, the roof of the tendon sheath can be opened out like a book, exposing the FPL tendon underneath.

Suture removal can be done on the same day. The POP slab needs to be retained for 3 weeks.
- At the end of 3 weeks, the POP is removed. If any K-wires have been applied, they are removed now. *The following are advised:*
  - Refer to physiotherapy for active mobilization of the fingers
  - Daily wash with soap and water
  - Massage of scar and grafted skin with coconut oil
- A compression garment must be applied to the operated fingers and maintained for a minimum of 3 months.
- Child is encouraged to continue the mobilization of the fingers; both active and passive and review once every month for evaluation.

Hypoplastic Thumb—Pollicization

51

Assessment (Hypoplastic Thumb)

Hypoplasia of the thumb can occur in varying degrees (Fig. 13.51.1).

- Grade I: Normal thumb, but smaller in size
- Grade II: Smaller than normal, weakness of the thenar muscles may be present
- Grade III: Short thumb with complete absence of thenar muscles
- Grade IV: Floating thumb—only a nubbin is present
- Grade V: Absent thumb.

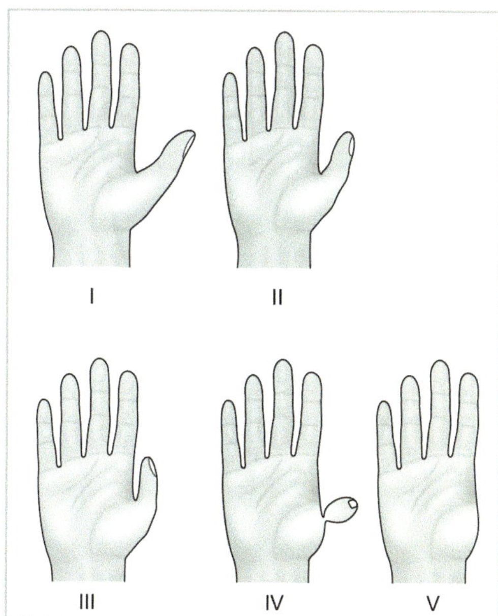

Fig. 13.51.1 Grades of hypoplasia thumb

In Grade I hypoplasia, no treatment is essential.

In Grade II, the individual case must be examined carefully to evaluate the function of the muscles moving the thumb. Appropriate tendon transfers will improve the function. In some neglected cases, the thumb web may be contracted. This must be addressed first, before any tendon surgery is planned.

In Grade III hypoplasia, the existing thumb may be too small to be able to do the normal work of the thumb even after tendon transfers. The option of pollicization may be considered to provide a working thumb.

In Grade IV hypoplasia, the floating thumb will not be useful. Hence, it must be excised and pollicization done.

In Grade V, total absence of the thumb, pollicization is a good option.

However, in all the conditions described above with pollicization as a treatment option, some parents may not prefer pollicization, as it entails removing the index finger and making it a thumb. If they prefer to add a thumb, the option of vascularized second toe transfer may be provided.

Pollicization

Presurgical Counseling

- This procedure will be done under general or spinal anesthesia.
- This procedure will take about 2 hours to perform.

fully before the next step is taken as there may be anatomical anomalies which should be identified and considered.

- There may be a common digital artery between index and mid finger. Along with the vessels, it is important to dissect the digital nerves too.
- *Flexor tendons and interossei*: The flexor tendons must be mobilized fully in the palm. The flexor sheath must be released from proximally, up to the base of the proximal phalanx (PPX) bone. Dissect the flexor tendons and the A1 and proximal part of A2 pulley. Divide A1 and A2 pulleys, so that A3 will become the A1 pulley of the newly created thumb.
- The palmar and dorsal interossei tendons must be elevated subperiosteally from the metacarpal shaft, taking care to preserve the neurovascular supply. Divide lumbrical at its insertion into radial slip of the dorsal aponeurosis.
- Elevate the first dorsal interosseous (FDI) muscle along with its innervation. The muscle dissected proximally up to the base of second metacarpal.
- Divide the two insertions of the first palmar interosseous muscle—into the ulnar slip of dorsal aponeurosis and into the PPX.
- Metacarpal bone.
- *Site of distal osteotomy*: Preserve metacarpal head of the index finger. Divide metacarpal bone at level of epiphyseal plate. The epiphyseal plate must be destroyed now by crushing.
- *Site of proximal osteotomy*: The second metacarpal bone is dissected. About 4 to 6 mm of base is retained. The bone is osteotomized at this level. The intervening segment of the second metacarpal is discarded.

Now, the finger is ready to be shifted. It will now be attached only by the following structures:

- Flexor tendons
- Extensor indicis proprius tendon
- Two palmar neurovascular bundles
- Dorsal veins
- Dorsal nerves.

Steps of Musculoskeletal Stabilization

- Step of skeletal readjustment
  - Position
  - The head of the metacarpal is now fixed in the position of the thumb (Fig. 13.51.4). This can be done by attaching the head of the second metacarpal bone to a point just palmar to the stump of the second metacarpal bone. It must be kept in rotation of the digit at about 140°. The new "trapezium" has been positioned now. But before fixing it, another point must be considered. The normal MCP joint of the index finger has got some hyperextension movements. This is not required when this joint becomes the carpometacarpal (CMC) joint of the thumb. Hence, to counteract this hyperextension nature, the head of the metacarpal is flexed and fixed in its position. The fixation can be done with a suture of 4.0 ethilon.
- Step of muscular realignment (Fig. 13.51.5).
- Now that the new thumb has been positioned and fixed, the muscular

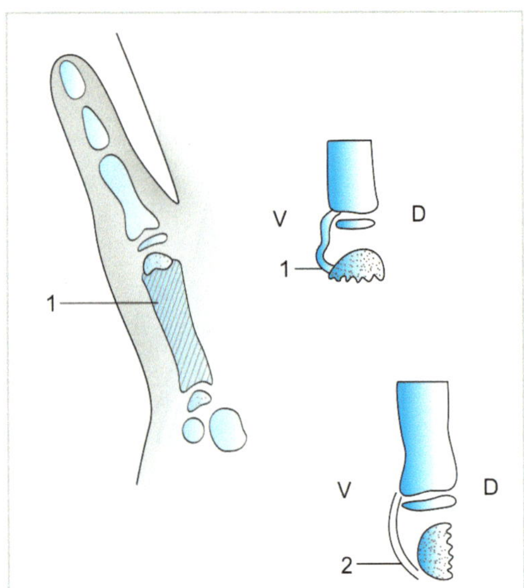

Fig. 13.51.4 Positioning the new carpometacarpal joint of thumb

Key: 1. II metacarpal bone; 2. MCP joint capsule; 3. V–Volar; 4. D–Dorsal

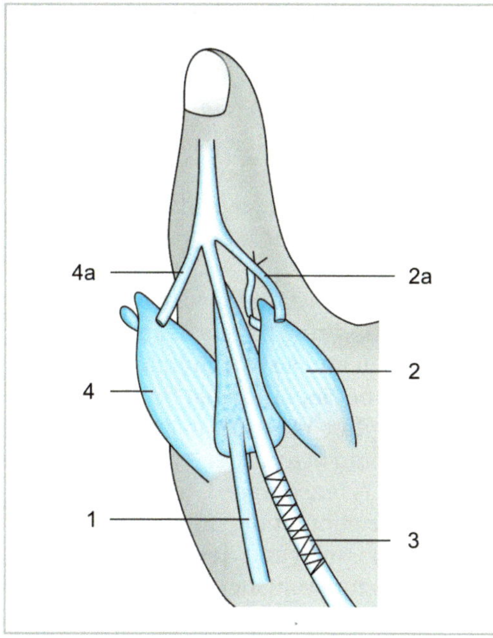

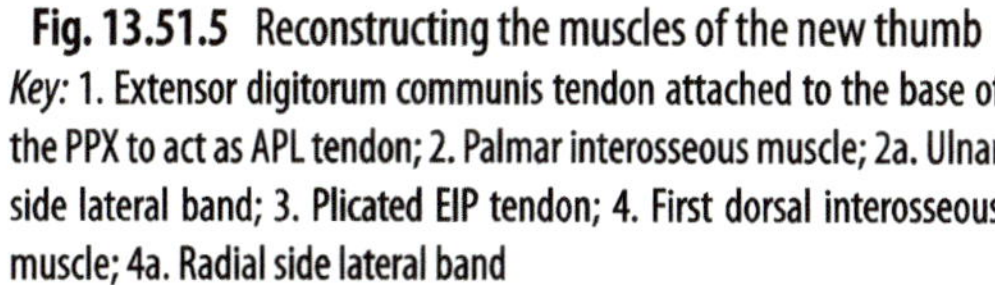

Fig. 13.51.5 Reconstructing the muscles of the new thumb
Key: 1. Extensor digitorum communis tendon attached to the base of the PPX to act as APL tendon; 2. Palmar interosseous muscle; 2a. Ulnar side lateral band; 3. Plicated EIP tendon; 4. First dorsal interosseous muscle; 4a. Radial side lateral band

attachments must be made. The long flexor tendons are already intact. The EIP tendon is also intact. With time, the flexors contract and act as a flexor pollicis longus (FPL) tendon. However, the EIP tendon will have to be plicated to help the thumb achieve a normal attitude.

- The radial side lateral band will be sutured to the dorsal interosseous to become the abductor pollicis brevis (APB) and the ulnar side lateral band will be sutured to the palmar interosseous to become the future adductor pollicis of the reconstructed thumb.
- The method by which this suturing of the tendons is by passing the free end of the cut lateral bands into a hole made in the musculotendinous junction of the respective muscles and suturing them back onto themselves with 4.0 polypropylene sutures.

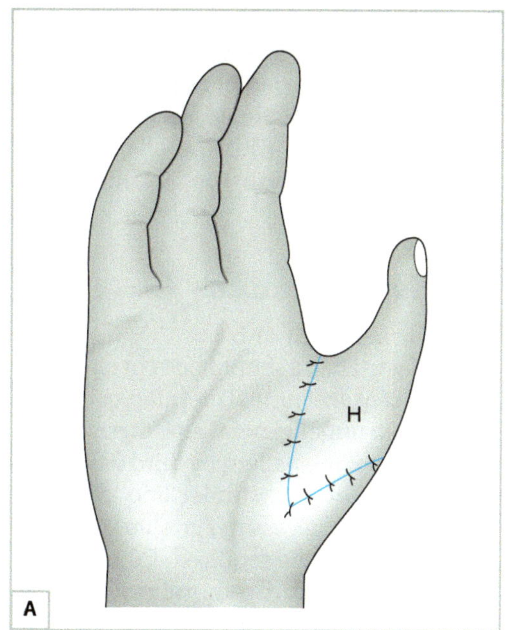

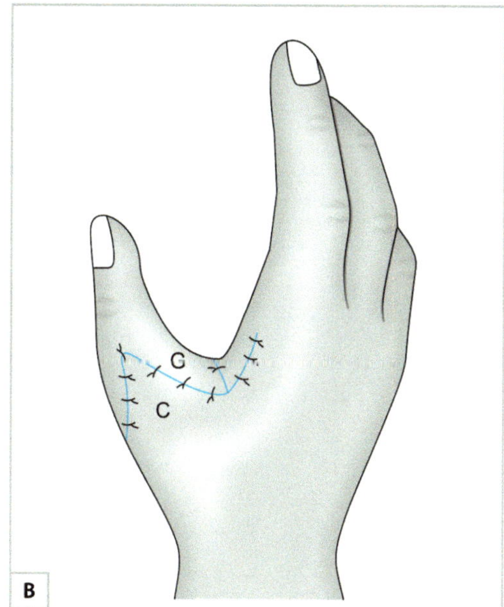

Figs 13.51.6A and B Final suturing of the skin flaps

- The tourniquet is released and the hand is covered with a saline gauze. The hand is kept elevated. Hemostasis is achieved and skin wounds sutured as shown in Figures 13.51.6A and B.

The hand and fingers are cleaned thoroughly and nonadherent dressings applied. Fluffy gauze pieces are applied between the fingers and sterile dressings applied. An above elbow POP slab is applied with the elbow in 90° flexion and the forearm kept in mid-prone position.

Postoperative Protocol

- Admission in the ward.
- The affected hand should be kept elevated.
- Patient can take normal diet after complete recovery if under general anesthesia.
- Discharge of the patient by third day.
- Inspection of the suture line after 10 days only. If necessary, a short general anesthesia may be required if the child is very anxious. Suture removal can be done on the same day. The POP slab needs to be retained for another 2 weeks.
- After a further 2 weeks, the POP is removed. *The following are advised:*
  - Refer to physiotherapy for active mobilization of the fingers
  - Daily wash with soap and water
  - Massage of scar and grafted skin with coconut oil
  - A splint must be applied to maintain the index and ring fingers in approximated position and a static thumb web spacer must be incorporated in the splint. This splint must be maintained for a minimum of a further 3 weeks.
  - Child is encouraged to continue the mobilization of the fingers; both active and passive and review once every month for evaluation.

SECTION

14

Common Clinical Conditions

Contractures on the Upper Limb—Assessment

52

Introduction

Contractures on the upper limb occurring as sequelae to either trauma, burns or congenital conditions form a major chunk of patients attending the hand surgery outpatient department in a developing country like India. Planning a treatment schedule for such patients is important, since rehabilitation is of immense importance. This chapter does not deal with conditions like Volkmann's ischemic contracture or intrinsic contractures, which are dealt in other sections.

When a patient presents with a contracture in any part of the upper limb, evaluation and planning the management is done based on various factors. The first criteria are the site of the contracture.

Examination of the Contracture

When there is a contracture on the upper limb, examination must show:

- Part involved
- Associated contractures
- Longitudinal extent of the contracture
- Quality of the skin over the contracture and the surrounding segment
- Nature of the scar—whether soft or hypertrophic, hyperemic
- Presence of any sinuses, ulcers
- Description of the attitude, position of the joints
- Active and passive movements of the joints
- Assessment of the apparent defect and the true defect.

In addition to the generalized examination steps outlined above, there may be certain criteria unique to some contractures, which will be described in the particular sections.

Contracture of the Finger

Additional Examination Criteria

- Involvement of the web spaces
- Involvement of the nail complex

Thumb

A thumb contracture must also be evaluated in the same way with a few points to be emphasized:

- Any associated thumb web contracture and measurement of thumb web angle
- Any associated bony problems.

Palm

Palmar contractures rarely occur alone, except in the rare condition called camphor burn, which is unique to our part of the country (India). Here, there is an isolated contracture on the palm, which may or may not cause a secondary contracture of the fingers.

The most important evaluation in a case of palmar contracture in the common criteria discussed above (points 1–8) is the estimation of the true defect.

Dorsum

Contractures on the dorsum of the hand very frequently involve the fingers and the thumb. Evaluation must proceed in the manner described above. In this site, assessment of the scar is very important, as it will decide the involvement of the underlying extensor tendons.

Wrist

The wrist contractures usually have underlying joint problems that must be corrected when the surgery is done. Hence, the evaluation of a wrist contracture must concentrate on the passive and active range of movements at the joint.

Elbow

Evaluation of elbow contractures is like the general evaluation of any contracture on the upper limb. Emphasis will have to be laid on assessing the quality of the normal skin around the contracture. This is because this skin can be used in reconstruction, when the contracture is released.

Axilla

Axillary contractures must be evaluated as critically as possible. This is because the release of the contracture must be planned based on the clinical evaluation. The examination of the scar will show whether the contracture is by bands of skin on the anterior axillary fold, or posterior axillary fold or involves the both folds of skin, and whether the axillary dome is intact.

General Examination

- Other contractures—neck, lower limbs, bilateral:
  - If neck contracture is also present, the management of the neck contracture gains precedence over the management of the other contractures. This is mainly for purposes of anesthesia, which may be difficult in the presence of a neck contracture.
  - If lower limb contractures are present, these also are more important than upper limb contractures, because with lower limb contractures, the patient may not be able to walk normally.
  - It is also important to note if there is a contracture on the opposite upper limb also, and the nature of this contracture.
- *Other scars:* Other parts of the body should be examined for presence of scars. This is important for two reasons:
  - Skin cannot be used from the scarred site when the contracture is released on the upper limb. For example, a thick hypertrophic scar on the abdomen may preclude the use of abdominal flap for resurfacing the defect after contracture release.
  - This scar also may have to be treated when the surgery is being done for the upper limb contracture.

Factors Affecting the Surgical Management

Age

In younger age group, the points to be remembered are:

- Skeletal growth is not complete, hence, a contracture when it is released, should be resurfaced with good skin that can grow with the affected part. Hence, the plan should be more for a flap cover than skin grafting.
- Even bilateral contractures can be released at the same sitting, since the patient will anyway be dependent on the guardian or parent.

- In planning a major surgery for a child, the probable blood loss should be estimated beforehand to avoid complications.

Associated Neck Contracture

If there is an associated neck contracture, this should be released at the first stage. No limb surgery should be done at the time of neck contracture release if it is felt that the blood loss may exceed the permissible levels or patient compliance may not be good.

Bilateral Upper Limb Contracture

Usually not released at the same sitting as this may make the patient totally dependent on his attender and this may prove difficult, especially for adult patients.

Contractures on Two Sites of the Same Upper Limb

When there are two or more contractures on the same upper limb, they are usually not

Table 14.52.1 Protocols for resurfacing after contracture release on the upper limb

Site of contracture	*Qualifying criteria*	*Plan of surgery*
Finger—single	Skin band contracture	Z-plasty
*Finger—single	Scar	Release and cross finger flap
Finger—multiple	Skin band contractures	Z-plasty
*Finger—multiple	Scar	Release and superiorly based abdominal flap cover
*Thumb	Scar	Release and inferiorly based abdominal flap cover
Thumb web contracture	Supple skin in web	Five flap release Square flap
*Thumb web contracture	Scarred skin	Release and groin flap cover
Palm contracture	Scarred skin	Release and superiorly based abdominal flap cover/pedicled radial artery flap cover
*Dorsal contracture	Scarred skin with mobile metacarpo-phalangeal (MCP) joints of fingers	Release and skin grafting
*Dorsal contracture	Scarred skin with fixed/subluxated MCP joints of fingers	Release and inferiorly based abdominal flap cover
*Dorsal contracture with thumb web contracture	Scarred skin with fixed/subluxated MCP joints of fingers	Release and groin flap cover
*Volar wrist contracture		Release and superiorly based abdominal flap cover
*Dorsal wrist contracture		Release and inferiorly based abdominal flap cover
Elbow contracture		Release and skin grafting
Axilla contracture	Skin band contracture	Z-plasty
Axilla contracture	Scarred skin	Release and skin grafting

* Indicates that adjuvant techniques will be required like:

released together because of the blood loss that may occur. In such situations, the release of contractures will have to be done one after the other.

Priority of Contracture Release

Proximal contractures should be released first. When the resurfaced skin—whether graft or flap, has settled well, and the full range of movements has been achieved at the released joint, the surgery of the next distal joint is undertaken.

Cause of the Contracture

If the contracture has been caused by flame burns, release of the skin contracture may suffice to achieve good function. However, if the contracture has been caused by trauma, or a congenital condition like flexion contracture, just release of the skin and resurfacing with skin tissue may not suffice, and good function may not be achieved without management of any underlying problem like tendon contracture.

Protocols for Resurfacing after Contracture Release on the Upper Limb

There are generalized protocols for resurfacing defects after contracture release. These protocols are not absolute and the surgery can be tailored to the needs of the patient (Table 14.52.1).

- *Bone surgery:* Arthrodesis of the interphalangeal joint of the thumb in severe contractures.
- *Joint surgery:* Release of the subluxated/ankylosed joint may be required in conditions like contracture release of the PIP joint or MCP joint of the finger.
- *Fixation with K-wire:* This may be required in conditions like release of a wrist contracture.
- *Muscle release surgery:* It will be required in conditions like thumb web release, where the contracted and fibrosed adductor muscles should be released along with the skin release.

53 Contractures on the Upper Limb—Management

Introduction

This segment on operative surgery will deal with the following surgical procedures only, since the other procedures mentioned have already been discussed in other chapters.

- Release of contracture
- Z-plasty
- Square flap method of thumb contracture release
- Five flap method of thumb web release.

Release of Contracture

The most important things to remember when a burn contracture is being released are the following points:

- Complete release of the contracture must be aimed at and should be the primary goal. Hence, return of function is prime.
- Excision of surrounding scar is a secondary consideration and should be contemplated only if total release of contracture has been achieved and excision of further scar will not compromise the hemodynamic status of the patient.
- Even if the primary plan is a contracture release and skin grafting, the surgeon must be prepared for a situation where there is an exposure of tendon or bone and a flap cover becomes mandatory.

The basic procedure for the release of a contracture is the same and the finer details are described here.

Surgical Steps

- First prepare the hand and the upper limb as described in the Appendix I.
- Marking the incisions:
  - The release incision should be marked on the contracture, in a transverse direction from one neutral line to the other. This pattern of release will reduce the chances of a recontracture.
  - At both ends of the marked incision, fish tailing incisions should be marked. These are "V"-shaped cuts extending medially and laterally from both ends of the incision. The length of these cuts depends on the amount of contracture release and can be extended, if release is not fully achieved.
  - If the scar is hypertrophic, like the dorsum of the hand and the elbow, tumescent solution can be injected under the scar in the plane between the normal tissues and the scar, to help in dissection (hydrodissection).
  - If the contracture is in areas like the axilla, where a tourniquet cannot be applied during the surgery, tumescent solution can be injected under the scar, to control the bleeding at surgery, due to the effect of the adrenaline component.
- The tourniquet should be raised and the surgery started.
- The skin incision should be made through the entire thickness of the scar, down to the subcutaneous tissue. Care should be exercised when incising thick, hypertrophic

scars, as the force required to go through the scar may be high, and the subcutaneous tissues may be injured in the sudden release.

- Once the subcutaneous tissue is reached, it can be identified by the presence of subcutaneous veins (especially in the elbow and wrist and dorsum of hand). On the fingers, these veins may not be prominent, but the yielding of the skin edges after incision, will indicate that the subcutaneous plane has been reached.
- Fibrous bands may sometimes be seen in the subcutaneous tissues. These should be incised totally or excised to achieve a full release.
- To aid in the release, the fish tail incisions as described above can be extended carefully.
- Full release may not be obtained in the following situations:
  - If there is a subluxation of the joint and a contracture of the capsule—here, the capsule of the joint should be released and the joint fixed with K-wires as necessary.
  - If there is a bony block or ankylosed joint, it should be osteotomized, the contracture released and formal arthrodesis of the joint should be done.
  - If there is a tendon contracture, like in the case of longstanding elbow contracture, where the biceps tendon gets contracted, total release may not be possible. In this situation, either the tendon can be lengthened by Z-plasty or the residual contracture can be accepted and dealt with later by wedging techniques.
  - Sometimes there may be a total release, but the joint may be springing back to the contracted position, like in the case of release of a contracture on the wrist. Thus, the released joint should be maintained in neutral position by means of a K-wire passed either obliquely or longitudinally.
- Once the release is complete, the bed of the raw area must be examined. If there is any area of exposed tendon or bone, a flap cover must be given as per the protocol described above. If there is no exposure of tendon, a skin graft can be planned to resurface the raw area.
- Apply wet gauze on the raw area. Raise up the hand and release the tourniquet. Maintain the hand in elevated position for about 3 minutes and ask for the tourniquet to be removed entirely.
- Now set the hand on the table. Assess the viability of the tip of the finger. It may take a few minutes for the tip of the finger to become pink. This is because of the fact that the vessels which were in a shortened length in the contracted finger are now stretched with the release of the contracture, and may hence go into spasm. If this occurs, apply xylocaine soaked gauze pieces over the vessels and wait for the spasm to be relieved. If the tip of the finger is still pale, remove any K-wires that have been applied. Wait for the viability of the tip of the finger to be confirmed and then secure hemostasis. Apply a wet pad over the raw area and prepare for the skin cover (whether skin graft or flap).
- The method of harvesting a skin graft has been described in Appendix VI. If a skin flap is planned, the flap may be raised as described in the relevant section.

Z-plasty

This procedure is done when there is no scar over the contracted area, but contracture bands. These bands have skin on their sides which can be redistributed to cover the area when the contracture is released. In executing a Z-plasty, planning is very important.

This procedure is ideal for contracture release of contracture bands on the fingers and axilla, where the joints are soft and supple.

Surgical Steps

- Prepare the hand as described in Appendix I.

- Markings for the procedure (Figs 14.53.1A and B):
  - Mark the ends of the contracture band as points "A" and "B". Draw the line AB. This line will run on the summit of the contracture band.
  - The contracture band will have two surfaces. From point "A", draw a line at an angle of 60° to line AB on one of the sides of the contracture band. This line should not cross the neutral line of the part. This means that this line should not cross the neutral line of the finger in a contracture of the finger and should not extend beyond the walls of the contracture band in the case of an axillary contracture. Mark the point where this line cuts the neutral line as "C". Measure the length of line AC.
  - Mark the length of AC on the line AB measured from the point "A". Mark this point on the line AB as "D". From the point "D", draw a line at an angle of 60° to line AB on the other side of the contracture band. This line, again, should not cross the neutral line of the part.
  - Thus, one Z-plasty has been designed. Thus, further flaps should be marked so that the entire contracture band AB is covered. Sometimes, it is possible that a single Z-plasty will cover the entire length AB.
- The tourniquet should be raised and the incisions made. First the summit of the band, i.e. AB should be incised. Then, the incisions should be made on the sides of the contracture band.
- Using skin hooks to hold up the tips of the flaps, they should be raised in the subcutaneous plane. When this is done on the finger care should be taken to avoid injury to the neurovascular bundles of the fingers.
- When the flaps are raised, apply wet gauze on the finger. Raise up the hand and release the tourniquet. Maintain the hand in elevated position for about 3 minutes and ask for the tourniquet to be removed entirely.
- Now set the hand on the table. Assess the viability of the tips of the flaps. It may take a few minutes for the tips of the flaps to become pink. Transpose the flaps to achieve the lengthening of the contracture band. If some confusion exists as to which flap goes where, just stretch the finger and the flaps will fall in place.
- Suture the tips of the flaps with 4.0 ethilon using the corner stitch (half-buried horizontal mattress). Suture the edges of the flap with 4.0 ethilon using simple sutures.
- Apply a paraffin gauze and sterile dressings. In case of axillary contracture release with Z-plasty, it is not necessary to apply a plaster of Paris (POP). In case of finger

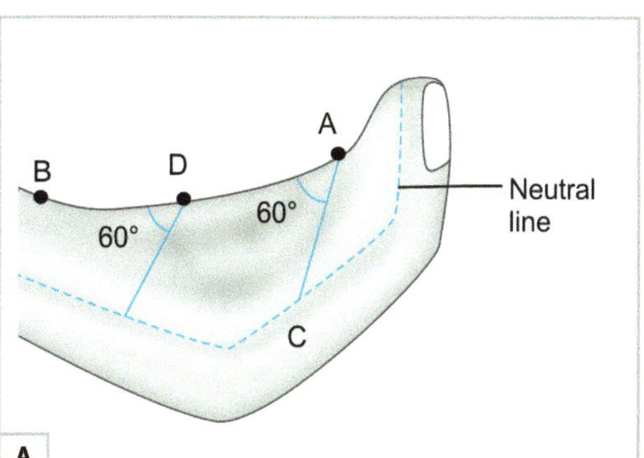

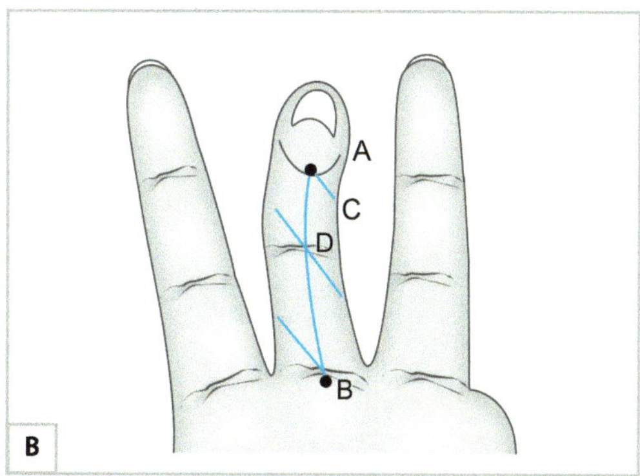

Figs 14.53.1A and B Marking the contracture release with Z-plasty on the finger

contracture release, a volar POP slab should be applied for the hand keeping the metacarpophalangeal (MCP) joints of the fingers in flexion of 90° and IP joints in extension.

Postoperative Protocol

- Admission in the ward.
- The affected hand should be kept elevated.
- Patient can take normal diet immediately if the procedure was under regional block or after complete recovery if under general anesthesia.
- Analgesics and antibiotics for 5 days.
- Sedation optimization strategy (SOS) for 1 day.
- Inspection of the dressing after 48 hours.
- Discharge of the patient by third day.
- Suture removal on the 10th day and removal of the POP slab and advice the following:
  - Refer to physiotherapy for active and passive mobilization of the fingers during the day
  - Daily wash with soap and water
  - Massage of scar and grafted skin with coconut oil
  - Straightening splints to the affected finger/fingers to be worn at night for a period of 3 weeks.
  - Compression garment for scar softening after a further 2 weeks.

Square Flap Method

This procedure is a preferred technique when a release of a contracture is required in the upper limb, especially a contracture of the thumb web or axilla. The requirement for this procedure to be done is a good quality skin on either side of the contracture.

Surgical Steps

- Prepare the hand as described in Appendix I.
- Markings for the procedure (Figs 14.53.2A and B):
  - Mark the ends of the contracture band as points "A" and "B". Draw the line AB. This line will run on the summit of the contracture band.
  - The contracture band will have two surfaces. From point "A", draw a line "AC" at 90° on one surface of the contracture. The length of this line must be equal to the distance "AB". Draw another line "BD" parallel to this line, from the point "B" on the same contracture surface.

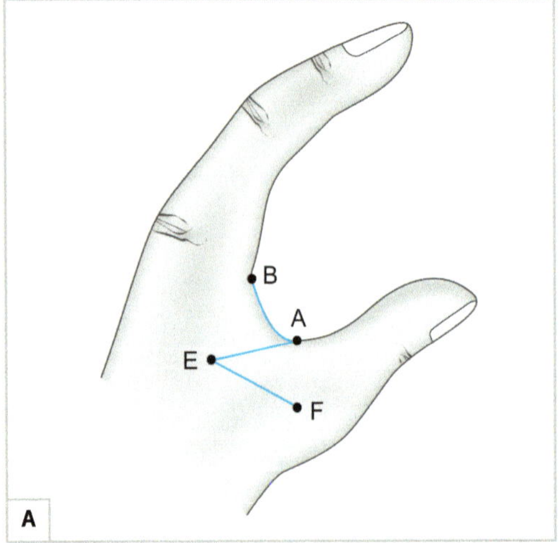

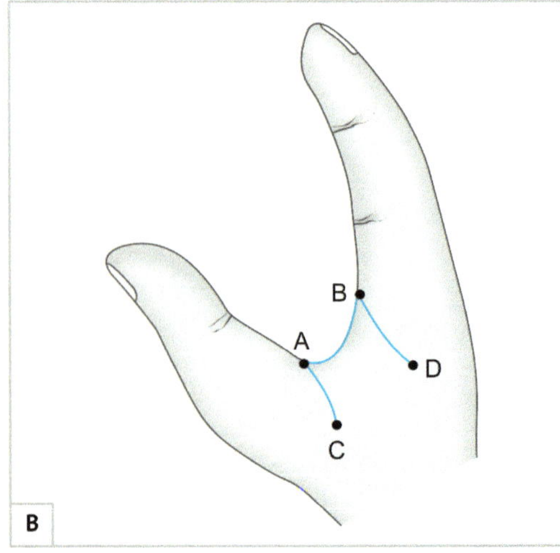

Figs 14.53.2A and B Marking the flaps

- Now the markings can be made on the other contracture surface.
- From the point "A", a line "AE" is marked at 45° on the second surface of the contracture. The length of this line must be equal to the distance "AB". From the point "E", another line "EF" is marked at 45° to the line "AE".
- Now surgeons have one square flap CABD and two triangular flaps FEA and EAB.

> When a contracture on the thumb web is released by this method, the square flap CABD is usually planned on the palmar surface of the contracture. The zig-zag flaps FEA and EAB are planned on the dorsal surface of the contracture.

- The tourniquet is raised and the surgery is begun.
- The incisions are made. First the incision AB is made down through the skin and subcutaneous tissues. The contracture will not get released by this incision alone. Now the incisions AC and BD are made through skin and subcutaneous tissue. Using skin hooks to hold up the tips of the flaps, they should be raised in the subcutaneous plane. When this is done on the finger or thumb web, care should be taken to avoid injury to the neurovascular bundles. Now the contracture will slowly start getting released.
- Now, the dorsal incisions can be made as follows. First the incision AE is made through skin and subcutaneous tissue. The flap EAB is raised holding the tip of the flap with a skin hook. Then the incision EF can be made and the triangular flap FEA is raised similarly. The flaps must be raised fully, based on the subcutaneous pedicles. When the flaps are raised, transpose the triangular flaps and advance the square flap as shown in the diagram. Thus, the leading edge of the square flap AB will get sutured to the line EF, the tip of the flap EAB will transpose and the tip "A" of this flap will get sutured to the point "D", and similarly, the flap FEA will transpose and get sutured to the point "C" (Figs 14.53.3A and B). Apply wet gauze on the raw areas. Raise up the hand and release the tourniquet. Maintain the hand in elevated position for about 3 minutes and ask for the tourniquet to be removed entirely.
- Now set the hand on the table. Assess the viability of the tips of the flaps. Secure hemostasis. It may take a few minutes for the tips of the flaps to become pink. Transpose the flaps as described above.
- Suture the tips of the flaps with 4.0 ethilon using the corner stitch (half-buried horizontal mattress). Suture the edges of the flap with 4.0 ethilon using simple sutures.

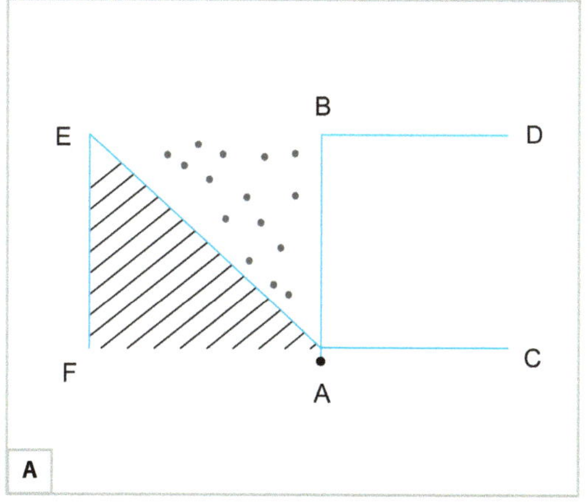

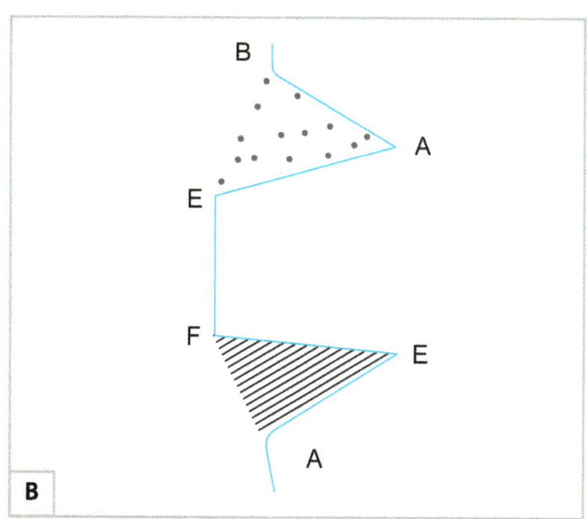

Figs 14.53.3A and B Principle of the square flap method

- Apply a paraffin gauze and sterile dressings. In case of axillary contracture release with square flap plasty, it is not necessary to apply a POP. In case of finger contracture release, a volar POP slab should be applied for the hand keeping the MCP joints of the fingers in flexion of 90º and interphalangeal (IP) joints in extension. In case of a thumb web contracture release, a good bulky padding must be applied over the freshly released thumb web and a volar POP slab must be applied with the wrist in 30° extensions, thumb kept in palmar abduction and the POP slab over the thumb web region.

Postoperative Protocol

- Admission in the ward.
- The affected hand should be kept elevated.
- Patient can take normal diet immediately if the procedure was under regional block or after complete recovery if under general anesthesia.
- Analgesics and antibiotics for 5 days.
- Sedation optimization strategy (SOS) for 1 day.
- Inspection of the dressing after 48 hours.
- Discharge of the patient by third day.
- Suture removal on the 10th day and removal of the POP slab and advise the following:
  - Refer to physiotherapy for active and passive mobilization of the fingers and thumb during the day
  - Daily wash with soap and water
  - Massage of scar and grafted skin with coconut oil
  - Dynamic thumb web spacer splints to the affected thumb web to be worn at night for a period of 3 weeks. In case of finger contracture release, finger straightening splints must be worn for the same period.
  - Compression garment for scar softening after a further 2 weeks.

Five Flap Method of Thumb Web Release

This procedure is a preferred technique when a release of a contracture is required in the thumb web. The requirement for this procedure to be done is a good quality skin on either side of the contracture. There are five flaps involved in this procedure. This technique is otherwise called a double opposing Z-plasty with Y-V advancement.

Surgical Steps

- Prepare the hand as described in Appendix I.
- Markings for the procedure (Figs 14.53.4A and B):
  - Mark the ends of the contracture band as points "A" and "B". Draw the line AB. This line will run on the summit of the contracture band. Mark the midpoint of this line "C".
  - Measure the distance AC. Mark a line "AD" equal in length to AC on one surface of the contracture at an angle of 60º. From the point C, mark another line CE equal in length to AC at an angle of 60º the line AC on the opposite surface of the contracture. Thus, two flaps of a Z-plasty (CAD and ACE) have been designed. Similarly mark two flaps for the segment CB as shown in Figures 14.53.4A and B. Since these Z-plasties are parallel Z-plasties and not in—series, care should be taken in the planning now. A line BF equal in length to CB is dropped at 60º from the point "B" on the same surface as the line AD. Another line CG equal in length to CB is dropped from the point "C" at an angle of 60º to the line CB. Now, two opposing Z-plasties have been designed and marked.

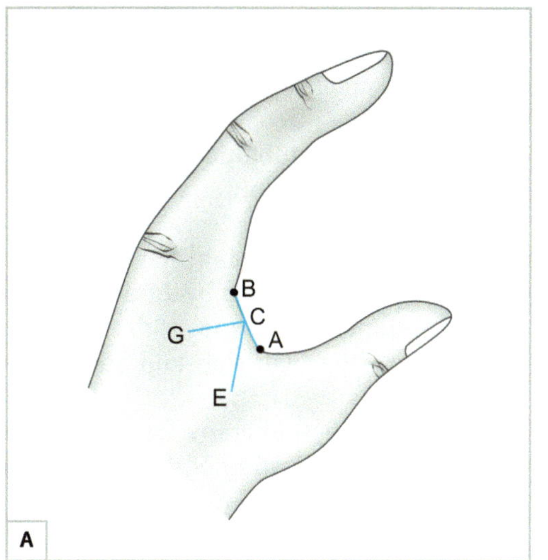

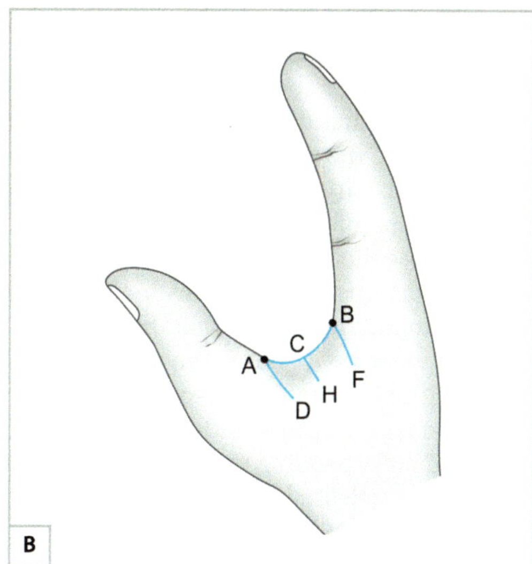

Figs 14.53.4A and B Markings for the five flap method

- From the point C draw a line CH equal to half the length of AC at 90° on the contracture surface where the lines AD and BF have been drawn. This line CH represents the "Y" limb of the YV plasty.

- The tourniquet is raised and the surgery is begun.
- The incisions are made. First the incision AB is made down through the skin and subcutaneous tissues. The contracture will not get released by this incision alone. Now, the incisions AD and CE are made through skin and subcutaneous tissue. Using skin hooks to hold up the tips of the flaps, they should be raised in the subcutaneous plane. When this is done, care should be taken to avoid injury to the neurovascular bundles. Similarly, incisions BF and CG can be made and the flaps raised as described. Now, the contracture will get released. The incision CH can be made.
- The flaps now transpose as follows (Fig. 14.53.5). The point "C" of the flap ACE gets sutured to the point "D". The point "A" of the flap DAC gets sutured to the point "E". Similarly, the flaps CBF and BCG transpose. The flap ECG advances and the point "C" of this flap gets sutured to the point "H". Apply wet gauze on the raw areas. Raise up the hand and release the

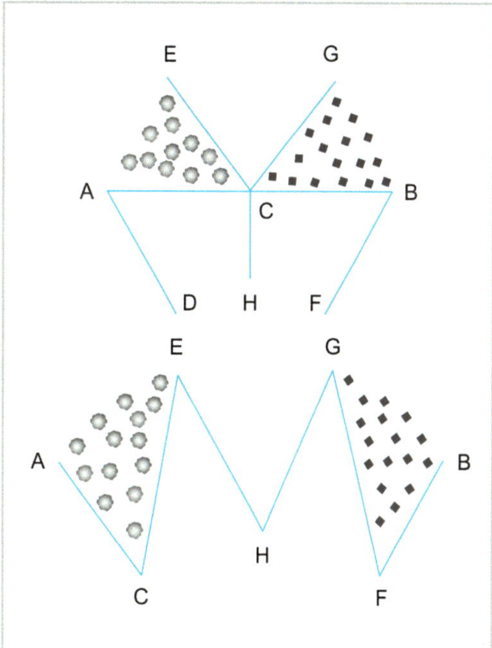

Fig. 14.53.5 Principle of flap movement in five flap method

tourniquet. Maintain the hand in elevated position for about 3 minutes and ask for the tourniquet to be removed entirely.

- Now set the hand on the table. Assess the viability of the tips of the flaps. Secure hemostasis. It may take a few minutes for the tips of the flaps to become pink. Transpose the flaps as described above.
- Suture the tips of the flaps with 4.0 ethilon using the corner stitch (half-buried horizontal mattress). Suture the edges of the flap with 4.0 ethilon using simple sutures.
- Apply a paraffin gauze and sterile dressings. A good bulky padding must be applied over the freshly released thumb web and a volar POP slab must be applied with the wrist in 30° extension, thumb kept in palmar abduction and the POP slab over the thumb web region.

Postoperative Protocol

- Admission in the ward.
- The affected hand should be kept elevated.
- Patient can take normal diet immediately if the procedure was under regional block or after complete recovery if under general anesthesia.
- Analgesics and antibiotics for 5 days.
- Sedation optimization strategy (SOS) for 1 day.
- Inspection of the dressing after 48 hours.
- Discharge of the patient by third day.
- Suture removal on the 10th day and removal of the POP slab and advise the following:
    - Refer to physiotherapy for active and passive mobilization of the fingers and thumb during the day.
    - Daily wash with soap and water.
    - Massage of scar and grafted skin with coconut oil.
    - Dynamic thumb web spacer splints to the affected thumb web to be worn at night for a period of 3 weeks.
    - Compression garment for scar softening after a further 2 weeks.

SECTION

15

Adult Brachial Plexus Injuries

Adult Brachial Plexus Injuries—Assessment

54

Introduction

When the patient presents at the outpatient department, surgeons aim is threefold and to identify the following three points:

1. What is the "level" of the lesion?
2. What is the "nature" of the lesion?
3. What is the "plan" of management?

Level of the Lesion

- Whether supraganglionic or infraganglionic
- Whether at the root level or trunk level or at any other level.

Nature of the Lesion

Is it a neuropraxia or rupture or avulsion?

Plan of Management

Once the level of the lesion has been judged and the probable nature of the lesion diagnosed, a plan has to be made for management. This should be a comprehensive plan, including the time of operation, the nature of operation.

All surgeons exercises for evaluation of the patient's condition, like clinical examination and investigations, will be aimed at the above three results.

Surgeons will go through the evaluation of the patient in a simplified way that will include clinical examination and investigations. At every step, surgeons will also see how it takes them closer to the aims of determining "level, nature and plan".

Clinical Examination

Clinical examination of adult brachial plexus injuries is given below (Table 15.54.1).

Motor Examination

Motor examination of adult brachial plexus injuries is described in Table 15.54.2.

Sensory Examination

Figure 15.54.1 shows sensory examination.

Investigations

Investigations of adult brachial plexus injuries are given in Table 15.54.3.

Documentation

It is very important to record the findings in a patient at the first visit. It is ideal that the subsequent evaluation be done by the same

Table 15.54.1 Clinical examination of adult brachial plexus injuries

S. No.	Parameter	Level of lesion	Nature of lesion	Plan of management
1.	*History:* Is it a low energy injury or a high energy injury?		A low energy injury usually will not cause rupture or avulsion, only varying degrees of neuropraxia and axonotmesis. A high energy injury will be likely to cause avulsion and rupture.	A neurotmesis or neuropraxia will require a waiting period to determine the spontaneous recovery.
2.	*History:* Is there any history of how the injury occurred—was the neck forcefully separated from the shoulder or was the arm forcefully abducted at the shoulder?	If the neck was forcefully abducted, it is most likely to have caused injury to upper trunks. If the arm was forcefully abducted, it usually affects the lower trunks.		
3.	*History:* Presence of severe pain		Deafferentation pain suggests avulsion injury	
4.	*General examination:* Look for other injuries: • Head • Spine • Lower limb trauma • Fracture clavicle			
5.	*General examination:* Shift of head away from injured side	Due to paralysis of paraspinal muscles-lesion at roots level	Likely to be avulsion injury	Poor prognosis
6.	*General examination:* Horner's syndrome	Suggests C8 T1 lesion	Likely to be avulsion injury	Poor prognosis
7.	*General examination:* Posterior dislocation of the shoulder	Avulsion at axillary nerve level		
8.	*General examination:* Palpable swelling in the supraclavicular region	Lesion of upper trunks	Most probably rupture—the neuromas are palpable	
9.	*General examination:* Tinel's sign at supraclavicular region	Lesion of upper trunks	If positive, most probably rupture—the neuromas are palpable. If no Tinel's, may suggest avulsion injury.	

Table 15.54.2 Motor examination of adult brachial plexus injuries

S. No.	*Action tested*		*Method of testing*	*Inference*
1.	Trapezius		Ask patient to shrug the shoulder against resistance.	
2.	Rhomboids		Ask patient to push both shoulders backward. Palpate the rhomboid muscles and compare between the two sides.	If working, means: • No avulsion • Rupture distal to roots.
3.	Serratus anterior		Push against a wall with both hands	Winging indicates palsy of the serrant
4.	Shoulder	Abduction	Keep elbow extended and move the arm away from the chest. Hold the lower end of scapula and note the movements here (rotation).	If not working, means: C5 involved.
		Adduction	Keep elbow extended and move arm toward chest wall.	If not working, means: C5 and C6 involved.
		Flexion	Patient stands with arm hanging by the side, elbow extended and fore-arm supinated. Ask him to move arm toward midline in front of chest.	If not working, means: C5 involved.
		Extension	Ask patient to do the opposite of the flexion.	If not working, means: C5 and C6 involved.
		External rotation	Patient stands with arm by the side of the chest, elbow at 90° flexion, fore-arm supinated, ask patient to move the extended hand outward.	If not working, means: C5 involved.
		Internal rotation	In the above step, ask patient to move the hand inward.	If not working, means: C5, C6, C7, and C8 involved.
	Elbow	Flexion	Ask patient to flex the elbow with the forearm supinated	If not working, means: C5 involved.
		Extension		If not working, means: C6 Involved.
	Wrist	Flexion		If not working, means: C6 and C7 involved.
		Extension		If not working, means: C6, C7 and C8 involved.
	Fingers	Flexion of flexor digitorum profundus (FDP) of index and middle fingers		If not working, means: C8, T1 involved
		Flexion of FDP of index and middle fingers		If not working, indicates C7, 8 involved

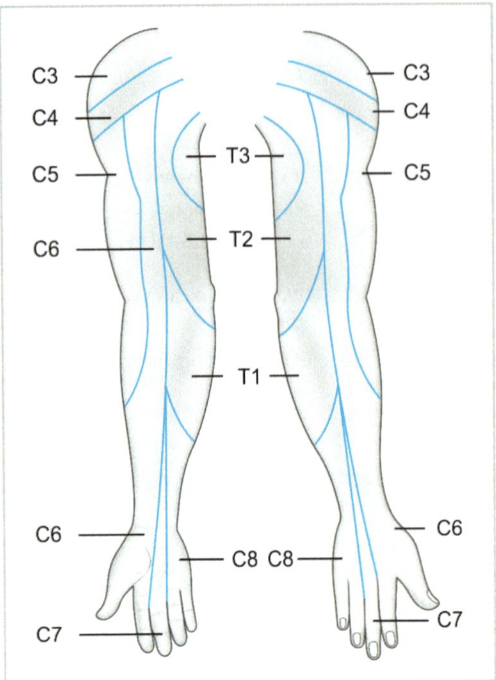

Fig. 15.54.1 Sensory examination

observer at the next visit. Hence, the record will help to chart the patient's progress.

See Appendix VI for the proforma that is routinely used.

Decision Making: What is to be Done?

Whatever surgeons plan to do must have the following aims to make the involved upper limb functional. And to do this, the following bare minimum must be achieved.

- Elbow flexion
- Shoulder stabilization
- Brachiothoracic pinch
- Sensation below elbow
- Wrist extension and finger flexion.

Now that the level of the lesion and the most probable nature of the injury have been made out, the decision to formulate the management must be made. Before making the decision, there are certain points to be remembered.

- If there has been a diagnosis of neuropraxia or axonotmesis, it is prudent to wait and keep evaluating the patient. A plan for surgery may have to be made in such patients as the findings warrant.
- If there is a diagnosis of avulsion or rupture, exploration of the brachial plexus is necessary as spontaneous recovery can never happen. Further procedure of nerve grafting or nerve transfer should be decided based on the findings at the exploration.
- It is very rare to have avulsion of all roots of the plexus in a single patient. Hence, there will definitely be some intact nerve which can be used for neurotization.
- If the surgeon is reasonably careful, exploration of the injured brachial plexus will not cause further damage.
- If there has been a paralysis of the intrinsic muscles of the hand, it is improbable that they can be made functional by surgery in the plexus. So, it is better not to do an exploration of the brachial plexus in such patients. However, an exploration can be done if there is associated pain, in an attempt to alleviate the pain.
- Contraindications for "exploration" surgery:
  - If the injury is more than 1-year-old, it may not be useful to do an exploration of the plexus and any subsequent nerve surgery in the plexus. After 2 years of injury, exploration of the brachial plexus is contraindicated.
  - If the patient is elderly.
  - If the surgeon does not have enough experience.
- Surgical plans when the patient presents more than a year after the injury or when the exploration and nerve surgery fail:
  - Muscle surgery
    - Latissimus dorsi transfer for elbow flexion
    - Free gracilis muscle transfer for elbow flexion, wrist extension, finger flexion
  - Bone surgery
    - Arthrodesis of shoulder if all the other procedures fail

Table 15.54.3 Investigations of adult brachial plexus injuries

S. No	Investigation	Significance
1.	X-ray cervical spine	Number of transverse process of vertebrae suggests injury at root level.
2.	X-ray chest—in inspiration and in expiration	To see function of phrenic nerve. If injured, suggests injury at root level, probably avulsion.
3.	X-ray shoulder	To look for dislocations and shoulder instability in upper trunk lesions.
4.	Computed tomography (CT) myelography	To look for pseudomeningocele if there has been an avulsion at root level.
5.	Magnetic resonance imaging (MRI) scan	Same as above, but visualization of the avulsed nerve roots is better.
6.	Electromyogram (EMG) studies: • In rhomboids • In serratus anterior • In paraspinal muscles	First check for activity in rhomboids and serratus: • If it is present, lesion distal to roots • If it is not present, check activity in paraspinals • If present in paraspinals, lesion distal to foramen • If not present in paraspinals, lesion proximal to dorsal ramus—probably avulsion.
7.	Somatosensory evoked potentials	

    - Should be done only if scapular stabilizers are intact.
- In our country, one more consideration—all patients do not come immediately and hence, the regular protocols may not be possible.
    - Priority wise—first attempt exploration and nerve surgery
    - Then, muscle/tendon surgery
    - Then, lastly, bone surgery.
- The results of nerve transfer are inferior to nerve repair.

Decision Making: When is it to be Done?

The plan has been made as to what procedure is to be done. Now, what remains to be decided, is, when to carry out the procedure. There are different time periods in which the different surgeries are planned.

- Immediate surgery:
    - When there has been a penetrating injury?
    - When there has been an iatrogenic injury?
    - When exploration has already been planned by the vascular surgeon for the subclavian artery, concomitant exploration and assessment of the brachial plexus injury can be done.
- *Waiting period:* If immediate surgery is not indicated, it is better to wait for a period of about 6 weeks.
    - If the patient has an incomplete lesion, it allows surgeons time to re-evaluate the progress of recovery
    - If the patient has a total palsy, the patient will have time to get all the investigations done and he will have time to experience the flail limb or disability.
- *Surgery at 6 weeks to 3 months:* It is the ideal period for exploration surgery to be done in patients with total or near total palsy? The period of inflammation is over and the tissues are soft and exploration will be fruitful.
- *Surgery at 3 to 6 months:* It is the ideal period for surgery for the following:
    - Partial palsy of upper levels

Table 15.54.4 Management protocol after clinical examination

Duration of lesion	*Findings*	*Plan*
< 48 hours	Penetrating injury associated with vascular injury	Immediate exploration
	All other lesions	Conservative management till 6 weeks to 3 months
6 weeks to 3 months	Total palsy Near total palsy	Exploration
	Incomplete palsy Partial palsy of upper levels	Conservative management till 3–6 months
3–6 months	• Total palsy • Near total palsy • Partial palsy of upper levels—with no recovery • Incomplete palsy with recovery only distal muscles	Exploration
	Other lesions	Conservative management
6 months to 1 year	Total palsy Near total palsy	Exploration
	Palsy of upper plexus	Distal intraplexal nerve transfers
	Incomplete palsy of lower plexus	Tendon transfers
> 1 year	Any lesion	Muscle transfer Distal nerve transfers
> 2 years	Neglected injuries Failures after surgical management	Bone surgery Tendon transfers

- Cases of incomplete palsy who have no recovery at all
- Cases of incomplete palsy who have recovered only the distal group of muscles over the period of 3 to 6 months.

Management Protocol After Clinical Examination

Management protocol after clinical examination is described in Table 15.54.4.

Adult Brachial Plexus Injuries—Exploration

55

Presurgical Counseling

- This procedure will be done under general or spinal anesthesia.
- This procedure will take about 4 hours to perform.
- This procedure is being done primarily to assess the injury to the nerves. The definitive treatment for the injury has already been made, but may have to be changed, depending on the findings that are seen.
- If the nerves appear to be intact, but surrounded by scar tissue, it is most probably an injury around the nerves. The scar tissue will be excised to release the nerves and recovery may be expected.
- If the nerves are found cut, they will be repaired. Recovery depends on the length of the nerve.
- If there is a gap in the nerves, it will be bridged with nerve grafts from the legs. Taking nerves from the legs will cause some loss of sensation on the lateral aspect of the sole of the feet. It will also cause a scar on the legs.
- If there is no nerve to supply the cut nerve as may occur when the nerve has been pulled away from the spinal cord, another nerve will be taken to supply the involved nerve(s). This will entail using a part of an intact nerve to try to bring back function to the affected nerve. By taking away a part of a nerve from another muscle will not cause any major deficit. The nerves that can be taken are the spinal accessory nerve or the intercostal nerves.
- Admission will be necessary for a minimum period of 1 week.
- Postoperatively, the affected upper limb will be immobilized in a sling and movements will be prevented.
- The result of this surgery will become obvious only after a few months of intensive physiotherapy and electrical stimulation and other supportive measures as will be required.
- During the period of physiotherapy, splints may have to be applied as considered appropriate by the surgeon/physiatrist.
- The general complications of general anesthesia can occur.

Position of the Patient

The patient is placed in the following position:

- Patient is placed in supine position on the operation table.
- A small pillow is placed below the space between the scapulae. This puts the neck in an extended position.
- The head is placed on a head ring. The head is turned to the side opposite to that of the lesion.
- The ipsilateral shoulder is depressed caudalward
- The anesthetist is requested to turn the endotracheal tube away from the side of the

lesion, so that the field for the surgeon and his assistant are free from protuberances.

Preparation

The surgical preparation is done on the neck, mastoid area, shoulder, ipsilateral chest and entire upper limb. The drapings are applied and the prepared upper limb is placed on the operation table, parallel to the patient's position.

Markings

- Segment "A" of the incision (for the supraclavicular dissection). The incision starts from a point just below the mastoid process. It then runs parallel to the sternomastoid muscle up to the junction between the middle third and lower third of the muscle. Here, the incision turns away from the muscle and runs parallel to the clavicle and runs about 1 cm parallel to it (Fig. 15.55.1).

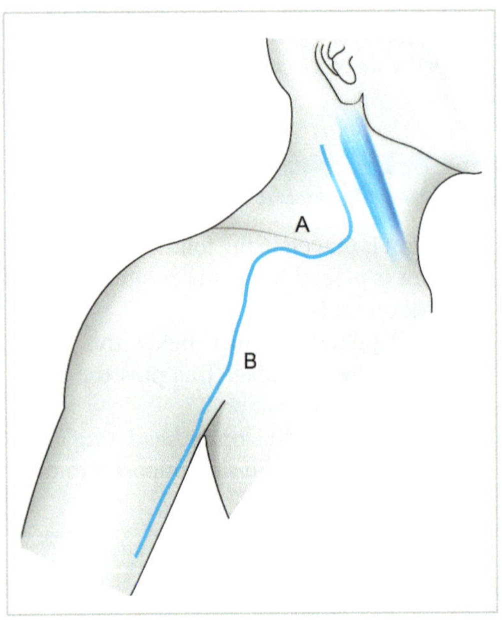

Fig. 15.55.1 Markings for the exploratory incision

- Segment "B" of the incision (for the infraclavicular dissection). At the lateral end of the clavicle, the incision turns downward over the clavicle at the level of the coracoid process to enter the deltopectoral groove. The incision then runs in the deltopectoral groove to the anterior axillary fold, which it crosses to reach the medial side of the upper arm. Here, it runs parallel to the brachial artery, up to the midpoint of the arm.
- It is not essential to make all the incisions that have been marked. The exploration usually starts in the supraclavicular area. If necessary, dissection can be done in the infraclavicular area.

Tumescent Infiltration

The markings are infiltrated with tumescent solution. The infiltration is done in the subcutaneous layer to control the bleed on making the incision. After a waiting period of about 6 to 7 minutes, the incision is made.

Surgical Steps

- Cross hatching marks are made on the markings and then the incisions are made. The incision is made on the sternomastoid region and the area above the clavicle. The incision goes through the skin and subcutaneous tissues.
- The next layer encountered is the platysma layer. This is also incised. Take care to avoid injuring the external jugular vein.
- So, now a flap consisting of skin, subcutaneous tissues and platysma is raised. It is anchored with 3.0 polypropylene.
- The sternomastoid muscle fibers are identified and the muscle is retracted medially to expose the superficial layer of the cervical fascia. This fascia is incised.
- Now, the following structure is seen—the cervical fat pad. Dissection in this area will

reveal the omohyoid muscle. This muscle is divided. The fat pad is retracted downward to reveal the underlying structures.

- First the transverse cervical artery will be seen along with its venae comitantes. This must be ligated. The deep layer of the cervical fascia is seen and now opened.
- The scalene muscles (Fig. 15.55.2) will be seen in the medial border of the exposed area. This can be confirmed by the presence of the phrenic nerve running on the surface of the anterior scalene muscle. These are retracted medially to further enhance the exposure of the area for the brachial plexus. The first structure that should be identified now is the superior trunk, either directly, or after identifying the C5 root.
- The roots of the plexus should be identified now. This can be done in one of the following methods.
  - If there has not been much scarring, the superior trunk of the plexus will be seen in the center of the exposed field.
  - If there has been some scarring, and the superior trunk is not easily visualized, identify the phrenic nerve again and then, this can be traced proximally to find the root of the C5.
  - Alternatively, the cervical rami which exit from the posterior border of the sternomastoid muscle can be traced

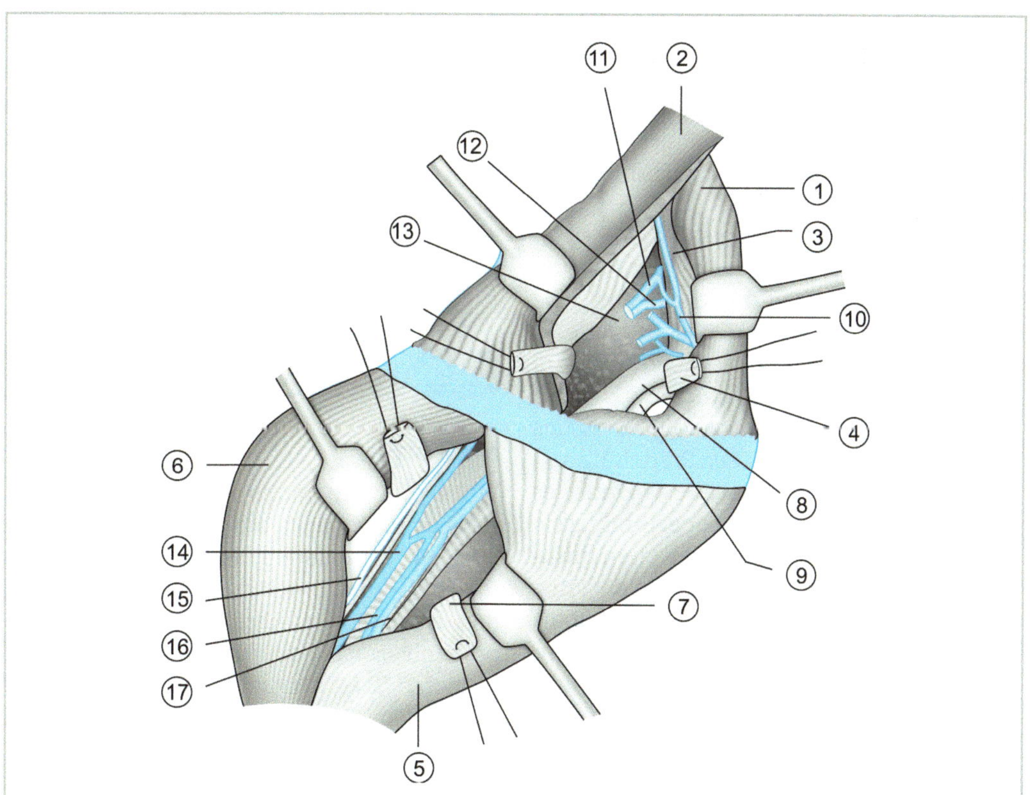

Fig. 15.55.2 Relevant anatomy on brachial plexus exploration

Key: 1. Sternomastoid muscle; 2. Trapezius muscle; 3. Scalenus anterior muscle; 4. Divided omohyoid muscle; 5. Clavicular fibers of pectoralis major muscle; 6. Deltoid muscle; 7. Divided pectoralis minor muscle; 8. Subclavian artery; 9. Subclavian vein; 10. Phrenic nerve; 11. C5 root; 12. C6 root; 13. C7 root; 14. Median nerve; 15. Musculocutaneous nerve; 16. Ulnar nerve; 17. Brachial artery

proximally to find the C4 root. This will serve as a guide to identify C5 root also.
    - If the C5 root has been avulsed, the root will not be seen. It will be lying near the clavicular area.
    - If C5 root has been identified, next the C6 root should be looked for immediately inferior and posterior to C5 root.
    - The C7 root is inferior to C6 root and is related to the transverse cervical artery.
    - The C8 root is inferior to C7 root.
    - The T1 root is identified immediately posterior to the subclavian artery.
- The anatomical identification of the trunks and divisions can be made in this dissection field itself. The avulsed segments of the upper roots will be found in the area behind the clavicle. The distal segments of ruptured upper trunks will also be found at this level only.
- The Erb's point can be identified by the three "divisions": (1) the suprascapular nerve, (2) the anterior division of the superior trunk and (3) the posterior division of the superior trunk.
- If the distal segments of the avulsed of ruptured roots cannot be seen in the surgical exposure afforded till now, the infraclavicular extension must be made.
- The incision is made as described (segment "B") of the marking. The incision is made through the skin and subcutaneous tissues down to the groove between the deltoid and pectoralis major muscles. The two muscles are separated and the clavipectoral fascia is reached. This is divided and when this is done, it may be necessary to divide some of the fibers of insertion of the pectoralis major muscle also. Retractors are applied medially and the insertion of the pectoralis minor muscle is identified deep to the pectoralis major muscle. This will be just medial to the coracobrachialis muscle.
- The pectoralis minor muscle is dissected, and divided between clamps. Retractors are applied both medially and laterally and the infraclavicular portion of the plexus is exposed.
- Identification points for the structures seen at this level:
    - The lateral cord will usually be seen in the center of this field.
    - The medial cord will be seen inferior and medial to the subclavian/axillary artery.
    - The posterior cord will be identified easier on the posterior aspect of the subclavian/axillary axis.
- Now, the findings are noted. There are some characteristic findings that are described below:
    - The plexus may appear intact, but for some appearance of thickened portions which suggest a neuroma-in-continuity.
    - There may be avulsion; the roots may not be available at the foramina and the avulsed segments may be lying distally.
    - There may be rupture of the nerve segments; roots may appear intact, but on following them, there may be a loss of continuity.

The brachial plexus has been dissected and the findings recorded. Now is the time to make decisions.

Decision Making

Neurolysis

When on exploration, the nerve plexus appears to be intact, but evidence of scarring is seen at different levels, neurolysis is planned. This procedure aims at clearing the scar tissues around the plexus that are probably causing compression to the neural elements. This scar may be either around the plexal elements or within the epineurium of the nerves.

The process of freeing the plexus from the scar tissue around the nerves is called "external neurolysis" and the process of freeing of the fascicles of the nerves from the scar within the epineurium is called "internal neurolysis".

The technique of neurolysis is described in the Chapter on "Nerve Surgery".

Nerve Repair—Primary

When the exploration of the neck is done, the altered anatomy is studied in detail. When there has been an injury to the nerve or the cord, and there is no loss of tissue, primary repair is done as described in the Chapter on "Nerve Surgery".

Nerve Grafting

In the process of exploration, when loss of part of a nerve continuity is seen, it is ideal to reconstruct this defect with a nerve graft. As discussed earlier, the primary requirements before doing a nerve graft procedure are:

- A good source of nerve to grow into the graft. The donor nerve that is available should be of good quantity and quality.
- A good nerve graft source that can be used without any residual morbidity.

Sources of grafts:

- *Sural nerve:* Most commonly used nerve graft source.
- Medial/lateral cutaneous nerve of arm and forearm
- Superficial radial cutaneous nerve
- Lateral femoral nerve
- Superficial peroneal nerve/saphenous nerve
- Split/whole ulnar nerve.
- Good conditions for the growth of the nerve into the graft:
- The length of the defect should not be more than 10 cm. This is because a graft more than 10 cm long will be nonvascularized and hence the recovery will be poor. In such situations, there are two choices available:
  - A vascularized nerve grafting can be done.
  - A nerve transfer can be done to avoid a grafting.
  - The bed of the grafting area should be free of scar and hematoma. Hemostasis should be perfect.
  - The duration of the brachial plexus injury should not be more than 6 months, in which case, the rate of growth of the nerve in the graft may not be enough to achieve good resultant function in the upper limb.

The technique of suturing of nerve grafts is described in the Chapter on "Nerve Surgery".

Nerve Transfer

There are situations like the following, where, nerve repair or grafting cannot be done.

- Avulsion of roots.
- Multiple level lesions with no continuity of the proximal nerve segment with the spinal cord.
- Ruptured nerve in which the proximal nerve segment does not appear healthy, or is heavily scarred and cannot supply enough neurons.
- Delayed cases beyond 6 to 8 months, where the slow growth of nerve in a graft may not be conducive to achieving good function.
- Cases with long segmental loss of nerve (> 10 cm).

In such situations, it is ideal to achieve neurotization of the important nerves with another nerve that can supply neurons and hence achieve function. The prerequisites for nerve transfer are the following:

- A good source of nerve to grow into the graft. The donor nerve that is available should be of good quantity and quality. There should be no residual morbidity as a result of use of this nerve donor.
- A valid nerve into which the nerve must be attached, so as to get useful function. This is particularly important in multiple level lesions, when not all segmental losses are made good, but only the important nerves for achieving useful function. This is because the availability of nerve graft source is limited.

Good conditions for the growth of the transferred nerve.

- *A good source of nerve to transfer:* The following are the nerves that can be used

Table 15.55.1 Management protocol of adult brachial plexus injuries—exploration

Finding	*Characteristics*	*Plan*
All components of the plexus appear intact		Internal and external neurolysis
Part of the plexus ruptured	Both ends of ruptured nerve available	Primary nerve repair
	Gap between nerve ends	Nerve grafting
	Duration > 6 months	Nerve transfer
Part of the plexus avulsed	C7 ruptured	Intraplexal C7 transfer
	C7 also avulsed	Extraplexal nerve transfer
	All roots avulsed	Contralateral C7 transfer
	> 8 months	Distal intraplexal nerve transfers

to neurotize segments of the injured plexus. The sources may be from within the plexus like the ipsilateral C7 transfer or the Oberlin transfer. These are "intraplexal" transfers. The nerve sources may be from other areas like the spinal accessory nerve or intercostals nerves. These are "extraplexal" transfers.
- Accessory nerve transfer
- Intercostal nerve transfers
- Commonly used nerve transfers
- Ipsilateral and contralateral C7 transfer
- Distal intraplexal transfer(Oberlin)
- Cervical plexus
- Phrenic nerve
- Medial pectoral nerves
- Hypoglossal nerve

- Nerve into which the nerve graft must be attached—this usually depends upon the priority that is before surgeons. Generally, the following is the order of priority for the distal end of the nerve graft.
  - *Upper trunk:* To achieve shoulder and elbow stability and mobility.
  - *Lateral cord:* To achieve shoulder stability, elbow flexion and hand sensation.
  - *Suprascapular nerve:* To achieve shoulder mobility.
  - *Musculocutaneous nerve:* To achieve elbow flexion and hand sensation.
  - *Medial cord:* To achieve finger flexion.
  - *Nerve to biceps and brachialis:* To achieve elbow flexion.
  - *Median nerve:* To achieve sensation in the hand.
- Good conditions for the growth of the transferred nerve:
  - A healthy bed with minimal scarring, which can be achieved by ensuring careful tissue handling and perfect hemostasis.
  - Good technique of nerve anastomosis.
  - Use of the microscope and fine suture materials.

Management Protocol After Exploration

Management protocol of adult brachial plexus injuries after exploration is given in the Table 15.55.1.

Adult Brachial Plexus Injuries—Nerve Surgery

56

Spinal Accessory Nerve Transfer

The spinal accessory nerve is a good donor nerve readily available in the field of surgery. If the nerve is divided as far as possible, there is hardly any motor deficit. This nerve can be used in any of the following ways:

- To neurotize the suprascapular nerve for shoulder abduction
- To neurotize the free vascularized gracilis muscle transfer being used for elbow flexion and finger extension.
- It may also be used to neurotize other nerves like the musculocutaneous nerve, using long nerve grafts.

Surgical Steps

- First, the suprascapular nerve is prepared to receive the spinal accessory nerve. The proximal end of the suprascapular nerve is trimmed under the microscope. The fascicular elements are looked for. The nerve is further trimmed in increments of 1 mm till normal appearing nerve is seen under microscope.
- The spinal accessory nerve is now identified. The posterior border of the exposed field is now examined. The plane between the sternomastoid and the anterior border of the trapezius is dissected and the nerve looked for. When the nerve is found, it is first confirmed to be the spinal accessory, by stimulating with a nerve stimulator, and noting the contraction in the trapezius muscle.
- The nerve is dissected as distally as possible. It will be seen that there are many small branches from the main nerve to the muscle at different levels. These branches must be spared to avoid totally denervating the trapezius muscle.
- The nerve is divided as far as possible. The cut end is now brought to the prepared proximal end of the suprascapular nerve. There should be no tension between the two ends. If there is evidence of tension, some more mobilization of the nerves can be attempted by releasing them from soft tissues. If this maneuver is not successful, a nerve graft may have to be interposed between the ends of the nerve. The procedure of harvesting the sural nerve graft is described in Appendix IV. Usually, this will not be necessary, as the length of the spinal accessory nerve will be sufficient for a primary repair with the suprascapular nerve.
- Under microscope, the nerve suturing is done with 10.0 ethilon epineural sutures using simple interrupted suturing technique.
- The wounds are then closed after keeping drainage tubes.
- Sterile dressings are applied.
- A layer of padding is kept between the arm and the chest and the arm is strapped to the chest with adherent plaster. The elbow support sling is also applied.

Intercostal Nerve Transfer

The intercostal nerves serve as good donors of both motor and sensory nerves. These donors can be used in the following ways:

- To neurotize the musculocutaneous nerve for elbow flexion.
- To neurotize the median nerve for hand and finger flexion and sensation.
- To neurotize the triceps muscle to achieve stabilization of the elbow.
- To neurotize the free vascularized functional gracilis muscle transfer for finger flexion.

When it is decided to use the intercostal nerves to neurotize some elements, the third to sixth intercostal nerves are usually harvested.

Contraindications

The intercostal nerve transfer is not planned when there are multiple rib fractures or there is evidence of phrenic nerve injury as seen by elevation of the ipsilateral hemidiaphragm.

Surgical Steps

- At the point where the original marked incision crosses the anterior axillary fold, the incision begins (Fig. 15.56.1). It runs caudally, in the anterior axillary line up to the seventh rib. The incision then curves gently transversely along the lower border of the seventh rib up to the mid-clavicular line.
- The incision is made down through the skin and subcutaneous tissues and the flap of skin on the anterior chest is raised.
- The pectoralis major muscle is retracted.
- The neurovascular bundle runs on the inferior surface of the corresponding rib. The nerve is extraperiosteal.
- The nerve is dissected gently from the mid-axillary line distally along the curvature of the rib. The nerve is very thin and must not be held with forceps at any time during the dissection. Gentle retraction with a skin hook will be enough.
- The sensory branches also should be dissected and tagged.
- Cautery must be avoided close to the nerve.
- After the nerve is harvested, it can be grouped along with the other intercostal nerves (Fig. 15.56.2) that has been harvested and taken to the decided recipient.

Hemostasis should be achieved and wounds closed. Sterile dressings and dressing applied on the chest.

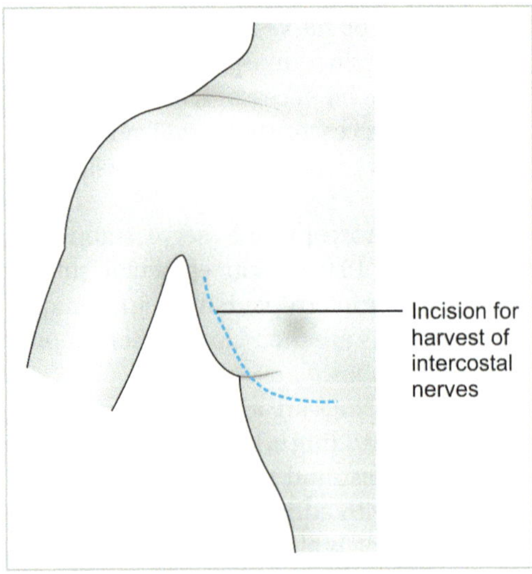

Fig. 15.56.1 Markings for the incision

Oberlin Transfer

The Oberlin transfer is a method by which a fascicle from the intact ulnar and median nerves are used to neurotize the biceps and brachialis muscles to achieve efficient elbow flexion. Obviously, this nerve transfer can be done only when the median and ulnar nerves are totally intact. Hence, this option is used in C5 and C6 lesions if primary nerve repair or reconstruction is not possible in the brachial plexus.

Presurgical Counseling

- This procedure will be done under general or spinal anesthesia.

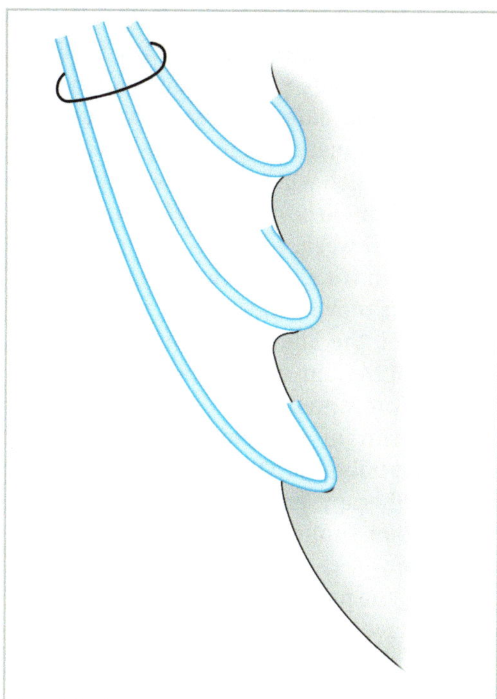

Fig. 15.56.2 Grouping together of the intercostal nerves

- This procedure will take about 3 hours to perform.
- This procedure will entail using a part of an intact nerve that goes to the hand to try to bring back function to the elbow. By taking away a part of a nerve from the normal nerve will not cause any major deficit.
- Admission will be necessary for a minimum period of 1 week.
- Postoperatively, the affected upper limb will be immobilized in a plaster of Paris (POP) slab and sling.
- The result of this surgery will become obvious only after a few months of intensive physiotherapy and electrical stimulation and other supportive measures as will be required.
- During the period of physiotherapy, splints may have to be applied as considered appropriate by the surgeon/physiatrist.
- The general complications of general anesthesia can occur.

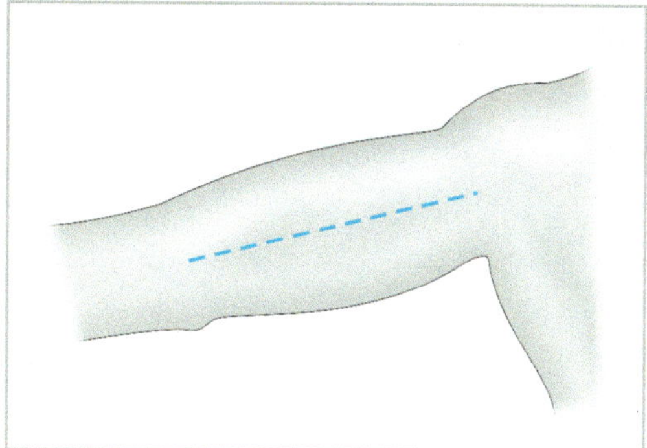

Fig. 15.56.3 Markings for the incision on the arm

Surgical Steps

Incision: It is made on the medial side of the arm in the middle third (Fig. 15.56.3). This is marked behind the palpated biceps muscle. This incision may have to be extended proximally or distally if it warrants.

Incision made through the skin, subcutaneous tissues and the skin flaps raised on both sides.

The biceps muscle is identified and retracted laterally.

- The brachial artery is now identified by the pulsation and will serve as a landmark for the identification of the nerves.
- The musculocutaneous nerve is closest to the biceps muscle. The branch from the musculocutaneous nerve entering the biceps muscle is identified and divided close to the hilum. The branch entering the brachialis muscle is also identified and divided.
- The ulnar nerve is dissected. At about the level where the nerve to biceps has been identified, the epineurium over the ulnar nerve is opened by sharp dissection and the fascicles are separated without causing damage (Fig. 15.56.4). The fascicles are stimulated individually to identify the fascicles going to the FCU tendon. These fascicles are divided and transposed to be coapted to the nerve to biceps. The coaptation is done with 10.0 ethilon or nerve glue. Similarly, the fascicles of the

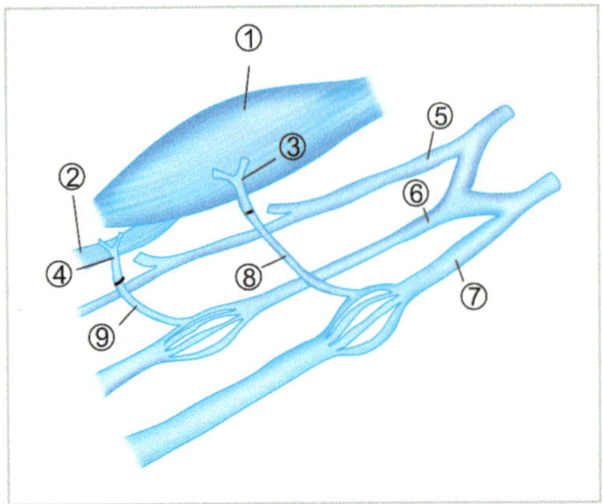

Fig. 15.56.4 Plan of nerve transfer

Key: 1. Biceps muscle; 2. Brachialis muscle; 3. Nerve to biceps; 4. Nerve to brachialis; 5. Musculocutaneous nerve; 6. Median nerve; 7. Ulnar nerve; 8. Fascicle from ulnar nerve; 9. Fascicle from median nerve

median nerve are separated at the level where the nerve to brachialis has been divided. The fascicles are stimulated individually and the fascicle supplying the FDS muscles is divided. This fascicle is transposed and coapted with the divided nerve to brachialis muscle.

- The wounds are then closed after keeping drainage tubes.
- Sterile dressings are applied.

A layer of padding is kept between the arm and the chest and the arm is strapped to the chest with adherent plaster. The elbow support sling is also applied.

Contralateral C7 Transfer

The contralateral C7 provides an excellent source of healthy neurons that can be spared.

Presurgical Counseling

- This procedure will be done under general or spinal anesthesia.
- This procedure will take about 3 hours to perform.
- This procedure will entail using a part of an intact nerve from the opposite side to try to bring back function to the affected side. By taking away a part of a nerve from the normal side will not cause any major deficit in that side of upper limb, except for some numbness on the index and middle fingers, which will improve with time.
- Admission will be necessary for a minimum period of 1 week.
- Postoperatively, there will be no restrictions on movements in the normal side. However, the affected upper limb will be immobilized in a sling and movements will be prevented.
- The result of this surgery will become obvious only after a few months of intensive physiotherapy and electrical stimulation and other supportive measures as will be required.
- During the period of physiotherapy, splints may have to be applied as considered appropriate by the surgeon/physiatrist.
- The general complications of general anesthesia can occur.

Position of the Patient

The patient is placed in the following position:

- Patient is placed in supine position on the operation table.
- A small pillow is placed below the space between the scapulae. This puts the neck in an extended position.
- The head is placed on a head ring. The head is turned to the side of the lesion.
- The anesthetist is requested to turn the endotracheal tube away from the normal side, so that the field for the surgeon and his assistant are free to work on the normal side brachial plexus.

Preparation

The surgical preparation is done on the neck, mastoid area, shoulder, ipsilateral chest and entire upper limb. The drapings are applied and the prepared upper limb is placed on the operation table, parallel to the patient's position.

Surgical Steps

The surgery consists of four components:

1. Harvesting the ulnar nerve from the affected limb.
2. Dissecting the contralateral C7 root and identifying the fascicles that are planned to be used as donors.
3. Coapting the vascularized ulnar nerve to the donor fascicles.
4. Planning the recipient nerves for the end organ neurotization with the distal end of the vascularized ulnar nerve.

Harvesting the Vascularized Ulnar Nerve

Incision: On the medial side of the arm (Fig. 15.56.5), extending distally behind the medial epicondyle on to the ulnar aspect of the forearm, up to the flexor aspect of the wrist.

The dissection is started in the wrist, where the ulnar nerve is easily identified.

Incision deepened through skin and subcutaneous tissues. Retraction of the FCU tendon ulnarward is done to expose the ulnar neurovascular bundle. The ulnar nerve is not divided until the entire length of the nerve up to the arm has been dissected.

The ulnar artery and the ulnar venae comitantes are identified and protected.

Dissection of the ulnar nerve is done, preserving the epineural covering and the blood vessels coursing in the epineurium. At the level of the elbow, the ulnar nerve is dissected in the cubital tunnel and freed completely. The nerve is then dissected into the upper thirds of the arm. The vessels running along with the ulnar nerve should be carefully preserved. Now, the nerve is tunneled to the opposite side neck by a subcutaneous tunnel created with a tendon tunneler.

Dissecting the contralateral brachial plexus and identifying the C7 root: The steps of this surgery have been described in the chapter on brachial plexus exploration. Once the C7 has been identified, it must be dissected as far as possible. The C7 divides into the anterior and posterior divisions. The anterior division contains the fibers for pectoralis major innervation. The posterior division contains fibers for neurotization of the latissimus dorsi muscle and triceps. These fibers can be used for transfer and will not cause any obvious deficit.

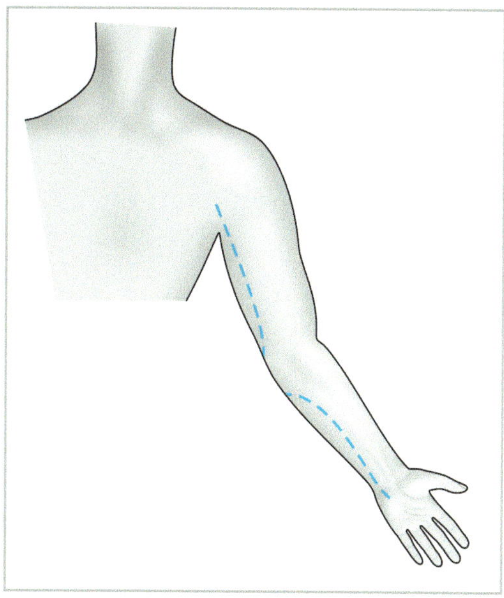

Fig. 15.56.5 Markings for the harvest of the vascularized ulnar nerve

Nerve suturing to C7 root: Distal end of the vascularized ulnar nerve is first tunneled across in a subcutaneous route to the neck incision on the contralateral side (Fig. 15.56.6) coapted with the selected fibers of the C7 root with 10.0 ethilon under microscope or with nerve glue.

Recipient nerve surgery: This can be done immediately or as a staged procedure. If done immediately, the recipient nerve is first dissected and kept ready. The recipient nerves are usually the musculocutaneous nerve, the nerve to triceps or sometimes to neurotize a functional muscle transfer, in which case it is done as a staged procedure.

- The epineurium of the ulnar nerve is carefully incised.

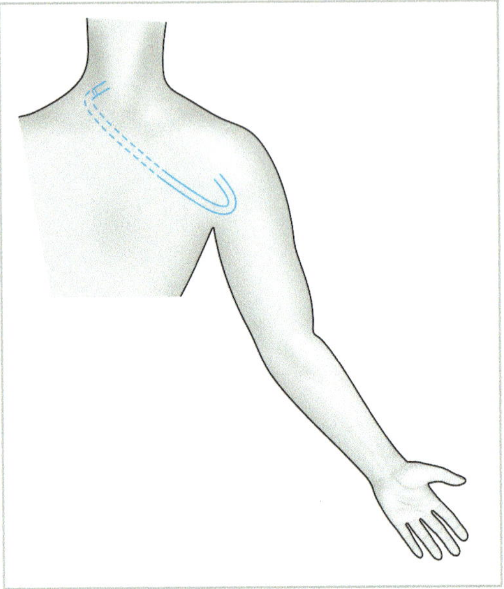

Fig. 15.56.6 Coapting the vascularized ulnar nerve to the donor fascicles

- The fascicles of the ulnar nerve are gently separated by fine sharp dissection.
- Nerve suturing done with 10.0 ethilon under microscope magnification.
- Skin wounds are sutures after securing hemostasis and drainage tubes are kept.
- Sterile dressings applied and arm restraint applied on both upper limbs.

Adult Brachial Plexus Injuries—Muscle Transfer

57

Pedicled Latissimus Muscle Transfer for Elbow Flexion

Presurgical Counseling

- This procedure will be done under general anesthesia.
- This procedure will take about 3 hours to perform.
- This procedure will entail using a muscle from the back to bring back function of flexion of the elbow in the affected side. By taking away this muscle, there will be no major deficit in the limb.
- There will be a scar on the back and sometimes a skin graft may have to be applied on the back, if it is not possible to close the wound.
- Admission will be necessary for a minimum period of 1 week.
- The upper limb will be immobilized in a plaster of Paris (POP) slab and movements will be prevented for a period of 4 weeks.
- The result of this surgery will become obvious only after a few months of intensive physiotherapy and electrical stimulation and other supportive measures as will be required.
- During the period of physiotherapy, splints may have to be applied as considered appropriate by the surgeon/physiatrist.
- The general complications of general anesthesia can occur.

Markings

Markings of the flap (Fig. 15.57.1) are made with the patient in sitting position, with arm held abducted at 90°.

- The posterior axillary fold is identified and an imaginary line is drawn to connect it to the posterior surface of the iliac crest. This represents the marking of the lateral border of the latissimus dorsi (LD) muscle.
- The midpoint of the axillary cupola is marked as "A". This represents the axillary artery in the axilla. Ten centimeter below this point along the lateral border

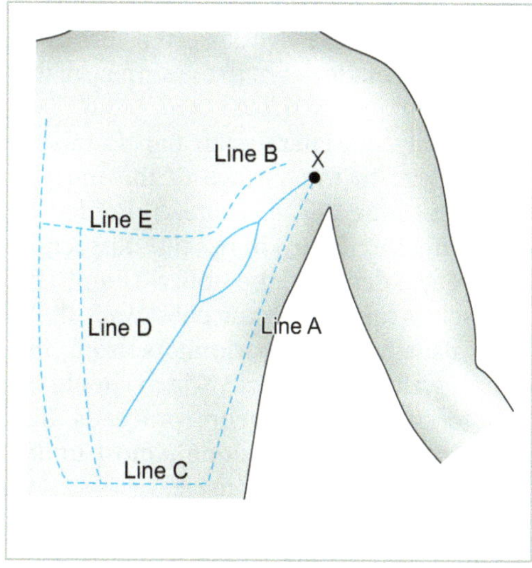

Fig. 15.57.1 Incisions for harvest of latissimus dorsi muscle

of the muscle is the point where the neurovascular bundle enters the muscle.

- A skin ellipse is marked about 5 cm × 12 cm, about 4 cm lateral to the marked border of the LD muscle and oriented parallel to the border. The cephalic apex of the ellipse is marked as "B". The caudal apex of the ellipse is marked as "C".
- Join the points "A" and "B".
- Extend the incision caudally for about 8 cm from the point "C", parallel to the lateral border of the muscle.

Surgical Steps

- The surgery is done under general anesthesia.
- The patient is placed in lateral decubitus position and the arm is kept in an abducted position.
- The entire back, neck, shoulder, half of the chest, entire arm up to the elbow is prepared and sterile drapings are applied.
- The incision is made first on the lateral border of the skin paddle ellipse. This incision is made down through the skin and subcutaneous tissues, till the surface of the LD muscle is seen.
- Now, the proximal incision "AB" is made only through skin and subcutaneous tissues. Then the caudal extension from "C" is also made down to the surface of the muscle.
- Now only the lateral skin flap is raised, superficial to the surface of the muscle. This is done till the lateral border of the muscle. From here, the dissection proceeds deep to the muscle, and the muscle is raised from the chest wall. There are usually many perforators from the chest wall to the muscle, which should be cauterized as the dissection proceeds. This dissection should be done almost under the entire span of the muscle.
- The lateral border of the skin paddle is now incised and dissected up to the surface of the LD muscle. Care should be taken to avoid dissecting between the muscle and the skin paddle. This can be ensured by applying stay sutures with 3.0 vicryl, between the surface of the muscle and the dermis of the skin flap. Now the medial skin flap is elevated over the surface of the muscle, till the origin from the paravertebral fascia. There are many perforators to the skin from the muscle, which must also be cauterized during the dissection. Now, the muscle is divided as far as the dissection limits.
- Now the vascular pedicle is identified. The vascular pedicle lies parallel to the lateral border of the muscle and runs 2 cm on the undersurface of the muscle. The branches to the Serratus anterior and Teres major are ligated and divided.
- Now the muscle has been totally dissected and is now attached only by the vascular pedicle and the tendinous insertion into the neck of the humerus.
- The tendon of insertion into the neck of the humerus is dissected and divided. The LD muscle has been totally raised on its vascular pedicle. The viability of the muscle and the skin paddle must be confirmed.
- The muscle is exteriorized and most of the incision is closed primarily with 3.0 polypropylenes after placing a vacuum suction drain in the wound and bringing out the free end in the mid axillary line.

Preparation of the Recipient Area on the Arm

- The patient is placed in supine position and the preparation of the arm is done.
- An incision "E" is made on the medial surface of the arm from the anterior axillary fold to the front of the elbow (Fig. 15.57.2). The incision is made through the skin and subcutaneous tissues and the atrophic biceps muscle is identified. The biceps tendon is dissected and isolated.
- An incision "F" about 5 cm is made transversely over the coracoid process. The bone is dissected and bared of periosteum.
- Now, the harvested LD muscle is now tunneled to the incision "E" on the arm.

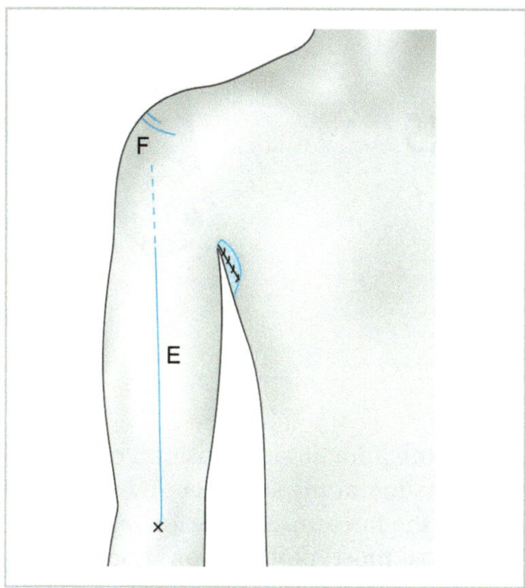

Fig. 15.57.2 Markings on the arm

Care should be taken to maintain the orientation of the muscle and care should also be taken to avoid kinking or torsion of the vascular pedicle. The viability of the muscle and the skin paddle must be confirmed again. If there is any problem in the muscle bleed, the vascular pedicle must be checked for signs of compression or torsion and corrected immediately.

- The tendinous insertion of the LD muscle must be oriented cephalad in the arm. This tendinous portion should be tunneled to the incision "F". Now, the suturing on the back can be completed.
- The tendinous insertion of the LD muscle must now be attached to the coracoid process to give a new origin for the muscle. This is done using 3.0 polypropylene with horizontal mattress sutures. Now, the incision "F" should be sutured with 4.0 ethilon.
- Now, the LD muscle is given a new insertion into the biceps muscle with 3.0 polypropylene. The elbow is kept in flexed position at 90° and the forearm is kept supinated.
- The wound is closed primarily except in the portion where the skin paddle is inset with 4.0 ethilon.
- An above elbow POP slab is applied with the elbow in 90° flexion and full supination. Gauze and pad dressings are applied on the back and the axilla.

Postoperative Protocol

- Admission in the ward.
- The affected hand should be kept elevated.
- Patient can take normal diet immediately if the procedure was under regional block or after complete recovery if under general anesthesia.
- The POP slabs must not be disturbed at all.
- Discharge of the patient by third day. Patient to retain the POP slab till the end of 4 weeks.
- Removal of the POP slab on the 21st day and advise the following:
  - Refer to physiotherapy for active mobilization of the elbow and fingers
  - Daily wash with soap and water
  - Massage of scar and grafted skin with coconut oil
  - To wear the elbow sling at all times for a further 3 weeks
  - Patient is advised to continue the mobilization of the fingers; both active and passive and review once every month for evaluation.

Obstetric Brachial Plexus Palsy—Assessment

58

Introduction

In a case of brachial plexus birth injury, it is not always that the hand surgeon gets to see the patient soon after the baby is born. Sometimes, it takes a few months before the baby is referred. In some instances, it may even take a few months or a year before the hand surgeon sees the patient. Hence, assessment of a brachial plexus birth injury must be accurately assessed at varying stages of the child's growth with the problem.

Eliciting the history is one of the first priorities in a case of brachial plexus birth palsy. Among the details to be found out are the following:

- *Specific antenatal history:* Whether there was occurrence of maternal diabetes.
- Details of the delivery—which include:
  - *Venue of delivery:* Whether in the hospital or at home.
  - *Method of delivery:* Whether by natural labor or cesarean section.
  - If by cesarean section, the indication, was it cephalo-pelvic disproportion?
  - If the delivery was by natural labor, was it a breech or cephalic presentation?
  - Was the labor assisted—with vacuum/forceps?
  - What was the birth weight?
- Attitude of the limb:
  - If the affected limb lies flail by the side and there is no movement at all, it denotes a total palsy.
  - If the limb lies in a position of internal rotation at the shoulder and pronation of the forearm, and flexion of the wrist, it is most probably an upper trunk lesion, which is the most common type of presentation.
- Signs of Horner's syndrome:
  - Ptosis
  - Miosis
  - Is evidence of avulsion of the lower roots and carries a poor prognosis?

The grading of the muscle power should be made and recorded. It may not be possible to test each muscle individually in babies and children. What can be tested are the muscle groups as mentioned below:

- Shoulder abductors
- Shoulder external and internal rotators
- Shoulder flexors
- Elbow flexors and extensors
- Wrist flexors and extensors
- Finger flexors and extensors.

Muscle Power Grading

- M0: No contraction
- M1: Contraction without movement
- M2: Slight movement with weight of arm supported against gravity
- M3: Complete movement against gravity.

Sometimes, the grading of the muscle power may not be possible. In such situations, and also in older children, it is

Table 15.58.1 Shoulder recovery (Mallet's classification) of muscle power grading

	Score = 1	*Score = 2*	*Score = 3*
Active abduction	< 30°	30°–90°	> 90°
External rotation	< 0°	0°–20°	> 20°
Hand to head	Not possible	Difficult	Easy
Hand to back	Not possible	Up to S1 spine	Up to T12 spine
Hand to mouth	Marked trumpet	Partial trumpet	< 40° abduction

ideal to classify as shown below. These tests are simple to perform and demonstrate to the child/baby. These positions can also be photographed/videographed for recording and assessment purposes.

Shoulder Recovery (Mallet's Classification)

Shoulder recovery (Mallet's classification) of muscle power grading is described in Table 15.58.1.

Elbow Recovery

Elbow recovery of muscle power grading is described in Table 15.58.2.

Investigations

- Nerve action potentials (NAP)
- Electromyography (EMG)

Table 15.58.2 Elbow recovery of muscle power grading

Movement	*Finding*	*Score*
Flexion	No contraction	1
	Weak contraction	2
	Good contraction	3
Extension	No extension	0
	Weak extension	1
	Good extension	2
Extension deficit (fixed flexion deformity)	0–30°	0
	30°–50°	–1
	> 50°	–2

Examination of the Baby at the End of 2 Days

This should be done in cases of total palsy of the upper limb seen immediately after birth. In such babies, after 2 days, there may be improvement seen and the real picture may be more apparent. This is because there is sometimes a conduction block immediately after birth, which is relieved by 48 hours.

Examination of the Baby at the End of 1 Month

The following are the types of findings:

- There is recovery evident in almost all the parts of the upper limb, like the shoulder, elbow and hand.
- There is absolutely no recovery at all, and this is usually the patient who has evidence of Horner's syndrome.
- There is recovery only in the hand function. There is no recovery of shoulder or elbow muscles.

Examination of the Baby at the End of 3 Months

The following are the types of findings:

- The biceps is recovering as evident by movements of flexion at the elbow.
- There is no recovery of the biceps.

If there is recovery of the biceps and shoulder muscles by the end of 3 months, recovery of the entire limb may occur. But, if there is no recovery, or there is only a recovery of the hand muscles, it is most likely that shoulder and elbow recovery will not occur normally. This is indication enough for exploration surgery and nerve surgery.

Obstetric Brachial Plexus Palsy—Management

59

Introduction

The surgical management of obstetric brachial plexus palsy consists of exploration and nerve surgery at the earliest. The procedure is the same as described earlier in Chapter "Adult Brachial Plexus Injuries of Exploration and Nerve Surgery".

Mod Quad Procedure

In obstetric brachial plexus palsy, muscle imbalances develop as some group of muscles overact and some muscles are paralyzed. This imbalance of action on the growing bones and joints creates deformities of which a few are common. When there is a palsy of shoulder abductors and external rotators, the shoulder goes in for internal rotation and adduction. With time, if this deformity is left uncorrected, the internal rotators and adductors—the subscapularis and pectoralis major muscle go in for contracture. If this happens, not only the child will not be able to actively abduct the shoulder, but even passive abduction also will not be possible. In such sequelae, the Mod Quad procedure is done which consists of four steps:

1. Release of the contracted pectoralis major and subscapularis.
2. Reconstitution of the internal rotators by attaching the muscle of pectoralis major to the distal cut end of subscapularis tendon.
3. Transfer of the latissimus dorsi muscle to supraspinatus for shoulder abduction.
4. Transfer of teres major muscle to teres minor for external rotation.

It is not essential that all these steps be performed for all the patients with obstetric brachial plexus palsy. Some children have good abduction, and no internal rotation contracture. But, they have no external rotation and this is a deficit that must be corrected. Hence, the surgery must be tailored to the need of the individual patient.

Presurgical Counseling

- This procedure will be done under general anesthesia.
- This procedure will take about 3 hours to perform.
- This procedure will entail using two muscles from the back to bring back function of flexion of the elbow in the affected side. By taking away these muscles, there will be no major deficit in the limb. There will also be a procedure done on the front of the shoulder where a release of the contracted muscles will be done.
- There will be a scar on the front and back of the shoulder.
- Admission will be necessary for a minimum period of 1 week.
- The upper limb will be immobilized in a plaster of Paris (POP) slab and movements will be prevented for a period of 4 weeks.
- The result of this surgery will become obvious only after a few months of intensive physiotherapy and electrical stimulation

and other supportive measures as will be required.

- During the period of physiotherapy, splints may have to be applied as considered appropriate by the surgeon/physiatrist.
- The general complications of general anesthesia can occur.

Position of the Patient

The patient is placed in the following position:

- Patient is placed in lateral position on the operation table with the involved side uppermost with the provision to make the patient in supine position during the early phase of surgery for release of the pectoralis major and subscapularis.
- A small pillow is placed in front of the chest, and the child rests on the pillow with a slightly pronated torso.
- The involved upper limb is placed in a position of abduction of 90° at the shoulder and elbow in 90° flexion with internal rotation of the shoulder. This limb is placed over sterile drapes applied over a hand rest.
- The head is placed on a head ring.
- The anesthetist is requested to turn the endotracheal tube away from the side of the lesion, so that the field for the surgeon and his assistant are free from protuberances.

Preparation

The surgical preparation is done on the neck, mastoid area, shoulder, ipsilateral chest and back up to the midline on the respective sides, entire involved upper limb. The drapings are applied and the prepared upper limb is placed on the hand rest as described above.

Markings

- Segment "A" of the incision (for the release of the internal rotators). The incision starts from a point just below the coracoid process (Figs 15.59.1A and B). It then runs in the deltopectoral groove caudally and cuts the anterior axillary fold.
- Segment "B" and "C" of the incision (for the tendon transfer). At the posterior aspect of the shoulder, two incisions are made. First the spine of scapula is palpated and above this spine lies the supraspinatus muscle. A transverse incision "B" parallel to the spine of the scapula is marked. Another incision "C" is marked over the posterior axillary fold, palpating the free margin of the latissimus dorsi muscle. This incision is made to dissect the insertion of the latissimus dorsi muscle.
- It is not essential to make all the incisions that have been marked.

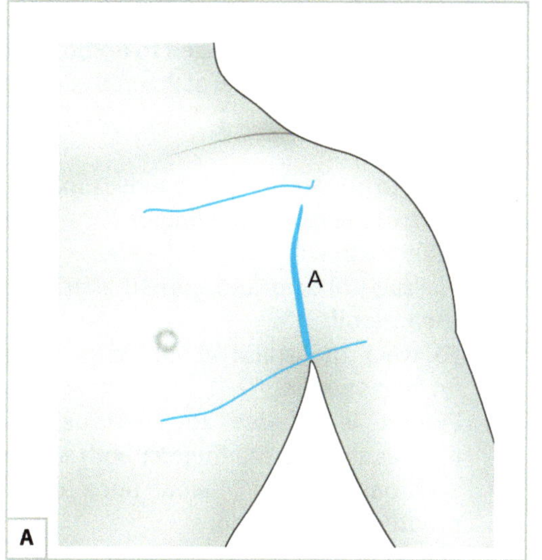

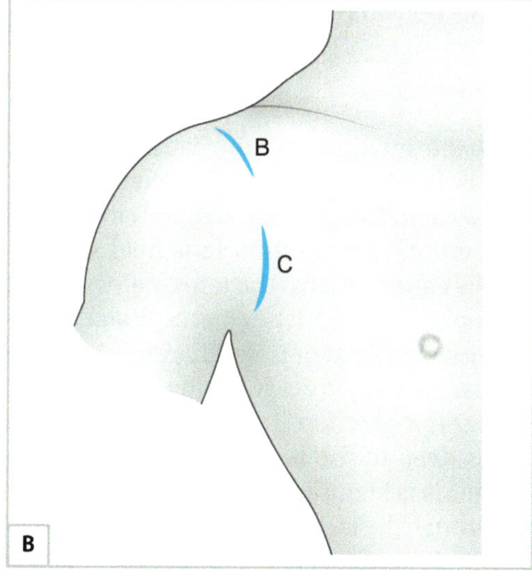

Figs 15.59.1A and B Marking of the incisions for the different components of the procedure

Tumescent Infiltration

The markings are infiltrated with tumescent solution. The infiltration is done in the subcutaneous layer to control the bleed on making the incision. After a waiting period of about 6 to 7 minutes, the incision is made.

Step 1

- Through the incision "A", the deltoid fibers are split and the pectoralis major muscle is identified. This is dissected distally to identify the insertion. The muscle is divided as close to the insertion as possible.
- Through the cephalad part of the same incision, the insertion of the subscapularis tendon is identified. This can easily be done by viewing the anterior aspect of the shoulder capsule. The tendon of the subscapularis is in the form of an aponeurotic sheet. This is divided proximally to retain as much of the insertion as possible. Now, passive abduction and external rotation of the shoulder will be smooth and free.

Step 2

To reconstruct the internal rotation, the divided pectoralis major muscle is sutured to the distal cut end of the subscapularis tendon with 3.0 polypropylene.

Step 3

- By the incision "C", the latissimus dorsi muscle is identified and dissected up to the insertion. The muscle is divided close to the insertion and the muscle is held with an Allis tissue forceps. The teres major muscle is now dissected. It lies just cephalad to the latissimus dorsi muscle. This muscle is also dissected up to its insertion and divided near the insertion. The teres minor muscle lies deep to the teres major muscle. This muscle is identified and dissected free.
- Through the incision "B", the supraspinatus muscle is dissected and the insertion is also identified.

Step 4

- The divided muscle of the teres major is sutured to the teres minor, close to the insertion, keeping the shoulder in a position of 90° abduction and external rotation. A subcutaneous tunnel is created connecting incision "B" and "C". The divided muscle of latissimus dorsi which is held by Allis tissue forceps is tunneled through this subcutaneous tunnel to reach incision "B". Here, it is sutured to the supraspinatus muscle close to its insertion.

Hemostasis is achieved and wounds closed primarily. Sterile dressings are done. The involved upper limb is immobilized in an airplane spline, with 100° of abduction at the shoulder and full external rotation, so that the palm faces upward.

Postoperative Protocol

- Admission in the ward.
- The affected hand should be kept elevated.
- Patient can take normal diet after complete recovery from general anesthesia.
- The POP slabs must not be disturbed at all.
- Discharge of the patient by third day. Patient to maintain immobilization of the upper limb in the POP slab till the end of 3 weeks.
- After 3 weeks, mobilization of the shoulder will be started retaining the POP. Hence, the child will be encouraged to abduct the shoulder above the level of the POP slab or splint.
- On the 21st day:
  - Refer to physiotherapy for active mobilization of the elbow and fingers.
  - Daily wash with soap and water.
  - Massage of scar and grafted skin with coconut oil.
  - To wear the splint at all times for a further 3 weeks.
  - Patient is advised to continue the mobilization of the fingers; both active and passive and review once every month for evaluation.
  - The POP slab will be discarded at the end of 6 weeks.

Volkmann's Ischemic Contracture—Assessment

60

Introduction

In our part of the country, Volkmann's ischemic contracture (VIC) is a condition that can be seen quite often in different stages of its development. The mainstay of the management of such a condition and attaining a good useful hand from a hand that has been affected by this condition depends on one main factor—correct and accurate assessment of the problem and the stages of involvement of almost all the structures of the hand.

Assessment of such a condition is aimed at:

- Determining the stages of involvement of the structures in the hand and the involvement of the structures that determine function in the hand.
- Determining the treatment plan which is basically dependent on the diagnosis.

Not all the cases of VIC that surgeons see will fall exactly into one of the types mentioned in Table 15.60.1. But, there will be a general trend that will categorize the type of lesion in a particular patient. As far as the treatment options are concerned, management will depend on the condition of the different structures in the hand (Table 15.60.2).

Planning the Sequence of Surgical Procedures

- *Physiotherapy:* As soon as the patient is seen in the outpatient department, especially if it is a mild type, the patient must be subjected to physiotherapy. This consists of mobilization of the fingers and splints to straighten out joints that are minimally stiff. This will even lengthen the minimally contracted tendons.
- *Exploration:* The first surgical procedure that is planned is usually an exploration. This procedure achieves the following:
  - It demonstrates the damaged structures.
  - It gives an opportunity to excise muscle infarcts.
  - The nerves can be assessed and the nerve surgery can be planned and done.

The timing of the exploration depends on the severity of lesion. In more severe types (Type II and Type III), early exploration is advised because it is important to bring back sensation to the hand. In mild type (Type I), the nerve is usually not involved. The exploration should not be done too early, as it may interfere with the healing of muscles after the trauma. Hence, this surgery can be planned after 6 months in Type I when the muscles have healed well.

- *Skin:* It is imperative that the skin on the forearm is of good quality and not scarred/contracted/adherent. If there are such problem scars on the forearm, they should be replaced with good quality skin cover as a preliminary procedure before embarking on exploration.
- *Skeletal problems:* Any deformities of the forearm bones or contractures of the joints must be corrected before planning any soft tissue surgery on the nerve or tendons.

Table 15.60.1 Type of lesions of different structures in the hand

Criteria to assess	*Type I*	*Type II*	*Type III*
Skin	Supple	Scarred	Contracture
Intrinsic muscles	Normal	Palsy	Contracture
Peripheral pulses	Present	+/–	+/–
Position of the wrist	Normal	Flexion	Flexion contracture
Position of the forearm	Normal	Fixed in pronation	Fixed in pronation
Position of the thumb	Normal	Simian thumb	Adduction contracture
Position of fingers	Flexion	Claw	Intrinsic plus deformity
Sensation	Normal	Loss of sensation	Loss
Finger flexion	Volkmann's sign	Weak flexion	Contracture
Fingers affected	Not all the fingers	All the fingers	All the fingers
Joints	Supple	Stiff	Stiff
Power of flexion of fingers	Good	Weak	Contracture
Power of flexion of thumb	Good	Weak	Contracture
Extension of fingers	Present	+/–	+/–

Table 15.60.2 Management protocol in Volkmann's ischemic contracture

Structure tested	*Findings*	*Management*
Joints	Stiff	Physiotherapy and splints
	Contracture	Arthrodesis
Skin	Thin skin Grafted skin Hypertrophic skin Skin contracture	Excision of the skin and skin flap cover
Flexor tendons	Good power one or two fingers only involved	Tendon lengthening
	Good power—only the flexor digitorum profundus (FDP) tendons involved	Tendon transfer: Flexor digitorum superficialis (FDS) → FDP
	Good power—all the fingers involved	Muscle slide operation
	Weak power not acting in Type II VIC	Tendon transfer: Brachioradialis (BR) → Flexor pollicis longus (FPL), extensor carpi radialis longus (ECRL) → FDP
	Weak power not acting in type III VIC	Free functioning gracilis muscle transfer for finger flexion
Nerve	Loss of sensation	Exploration and nerve reconstruction

- *Nerve surgery:* Restoration of the sensation on the hand is an essential requisite before contemplating reanimation procedures.
- *Joint:* The joints of the hand and fingers must be made soft and supple before any tendon surgery can be planned. This principle must be followed in keeping with the principles of tendon surgery.
- *Tendon:* The tendon procedures should be done after the other procedures are complete.

Examination of the blood vessels:

- The caliber of the radial artery and the ulnar artery must also be examined. The hand may already be viable, but it is ideal to have a good vasculature to the hand to ensure optimum healing of the tissues and function. If the vessels are obliterated, appropriate vein grafts to bridge the gaps and restore good blood flow to the hand must be done by microvascular anastomosis using reversed saphenous vein grafts from the leg.
- The tourniquet must be released and gentle pressure with a saline pad should be applied and the hand kept elevated for two minutes. Next, the hand must be placed on the table and hemostasis achieved. Skin suturing is done with 3.0 ethilon and drainage tubes kept in the proximal portion of the suture line. Sterile dressings are applied and dorsal plaster of Paris (POP) slab is applied with wrist in neutral position and fingers in position appropriate with the surgical procedure that has been done (nerve or tendon surgery).

Postoperative Protocol

- Admission in the ward.
- The affected hand should be kept elevated.
- Patient can take normal diet after complete recovery if he was under general anesthesia.
- Discharge of the patient by 3rd day.
- Inspection of the suture line on the 2nd day. If necessary, a short general anesthesia may be required if the child is very serious. Suture removal can be done on the 10th day. The POP slab needs to be retained for another two weeks.
- After further two weeks, the POP is removed. The following are advised:
    - Refer to physiotherapy for active mobilization of the fingers
    - Daily wash with soap and water
    - Massage of scar and grafted skin with coconut oil
    - Child is encouraged to continue the mobilization of the fingers; both active and passive and review once every month for evaluation.

Tendon Lengthening

Surgical Steps

- The involved tendon is identified and dissected.
- The excursion of the tendon is confirmed by a passive mobilization.
- It is divided with a No. 11 blade as shown in the diagram (Fig. 15.61.3).
- The suturing of the tendon is now done with 3.0 polypropylene, as shown in the diagram (Fig. 15.61.3).
- The tourniquet must be released and gentle pressure with a saline pad should be applied and the hand kept elevated for two minutes. Next, the hand must be placed on the table and hemostasis achieved. Skin suturing is done with 3.0 ethilon and drainage tubes kept in the proximal portion of the suture line. Sterile dressings are applied and dorsal POP slab is applied with wrist in neutral position and fingers in position appropriate with the surgical procedure that has been done (nerve or tendon surgery).

Postoperative Protocol

- Admission in the ward.
- The affected hand should be kept elevated.
- Patient can take normal diet after complete recovery if he was under general anesthesia.
- Discharge of the patient by the 3rd day.

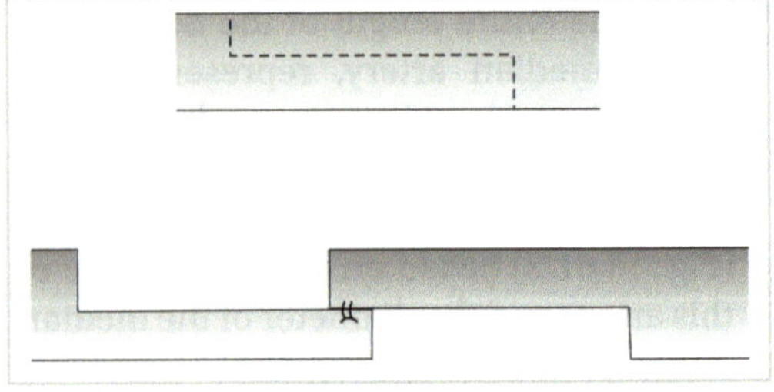

Fig. 15.61.3 Technique of tendon lengthening

- Inspection of the suture line on the 2nd day. If necessary, a short general anesthesia may be required, if the child is very serious. Suture removal can be done on the 10th day. The POP slab needs to be retained for another two weeks.
- After further two weeks, the POP is removed. The following are advised:
  - Refer to physiotherapy for active mobilization of the fingers
  - Daily wash with soap and water
  - Massage of scar and grafted skin with coconut oil
  - Child is encouraged to continue the mobilization of the fingers; both active and passive and review once every month for evaluation.

Muscle Slide Operation

Surgical Steps

- Incision on the forearm must extend from the wrist on the radial side to allow access to the flexor pollicis longus (FPL) tendon if necessary to the arm, proximal to the elbow joint.
- Identify the median nerve, which is just ulnar to the biceps tendon. Identify the brachialis muscle that is posterior to the median nerve. Identify the pronator teres muscle, which is immediately ulnar to the median nerve.
- Identify the ulnar nerve as it enters the forearm between the two heads of the FCU muscle. Palpate the ulna bone.
- Pass a retractor and retract to the radial side, the median nerve along with the brachialis and biceps. Pass another retractor to retract the pronator teres ulnarward. Palpate the medial epicondyle of the humerus in the valley between the two retractors. Incise the periosteum, and with a periosteal elevator, release the pronator and flexors muscle origin from the epicondyle, subperiosteally. This can be done from the radial side toward the ulnar side. It will have to stop when the ulnar nerve is encountered.
- Now, make incision on the ulna for the distance of the origin of the FCU muscle. Raise the FCU muscle subperiosteally. The ulnar nerve is still seen entering the FCU muscle. This need not be disturbed. As the FCU muscle is being erased from its origin, the ulnar nerve can be brought anterior to the medial epicondyle, to reduce the tension on the nerve. As this is being done, the elbow joint capsule and the tuberosity of the ulna will get exposed. When this procedure is done carefully, the muscle will be erased along with the periosteum.
- After the FCU is raised from the ulna, the interosseous membrane comes into view and the anterior interosseous artery, and its perforating branches and nerve and veins will be seen. These must be protected.
- Gentle traction must be given on the fingers to extend them. As the muscles are being released, the fingers will be able to be passively extended. The end point of this muscle elevation is the full, free passive extension of all the fingers and thumb.
- The thumb may not get released by the procedure described above. From the middle and distal segments of the incision, the FPL muscle is exposed and released subperiosteally from the radius to achieve full extension of the thumb.
- Now, the ulnar and median nerves must be released from all scars distally also.
- The tourniquet must be released and gentle pressure with a saline pad should be applied and the hand kept elevated for two minutes. Next, the hand must be placed on the table and hemostasis achieved. Skin suturing is done with 3.0 ethilon and drainage tubes kept in the proximal portion of the suture line. Sterile dressings are applied and dorsal POP slab is applied with wrist in neutral position and fingers in position appropriate with the surgical procedure that has been done (nerve or tendon surgery).

Postoperative Protocol

- Admission in the ward.
- The affected hand should be kept elevated.

- Patient can take normal diet after complete recovery if he was under general anesthesia.
- Discharge of the patient by the 3rd day.
- Inspection of the suture line on the 2nd day. If necessary, a short general anesthesia may be required if the child is very serious. Suture removal can be done on the 10th day. The POP slab needs to be retained for another two weeks.
- After further two weeks, the POP is removed. The following are advised:
  - Refer to physiotherapy for active mobilization of the fingers.
  - Daily wash with soap and water.
  - Massage of scar and grafted skin with coconut oil.
  - Child is encouraged to continue the mobilization of the fingers; both active and passive and review once every month for evaluation.

Tendon Transfer—FDS to FDP

Surgical Steps

Through the exposure described above, the following steps are carried out (Figs 15.61.4A and B).

- The FDS tendons of all the fingers are identified and dissected. The FDP tendons to all the fingers are identified and dissected.
- The FDS tendons are divided as distally as possible in the palm at Zone III level for all the fingers. The FDP tendons are divided close to the musculotendinous junction for all the fingers.
- The excursion of the FDP tendons is confirmed by passive mobilization. The proximal FDS tendon of the index finger and the distal FDP tendon of the finger are now kept in proximity. They cannot be sutured directly as the tension has not yet been adjusted. Too tight suturing or too loose suturing will result in a useless finger. The method of adjusting the tension is as follows:
  - The wrist is kept in neutral position. The FDS muscle is now going to move the FDP tendon of the corresponding finger. The proximal FDS tendon is pulled and relaxed alternatively to confirm the supple muscle. The distal cut end of the FDP tendon is also moved passively to confirm that there are no adhesions distally.
  - With the wrist in neutral position, the distal FDP tendon of the index finger

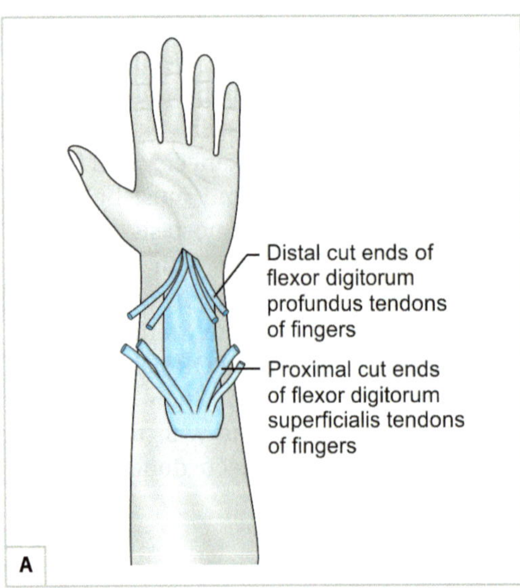

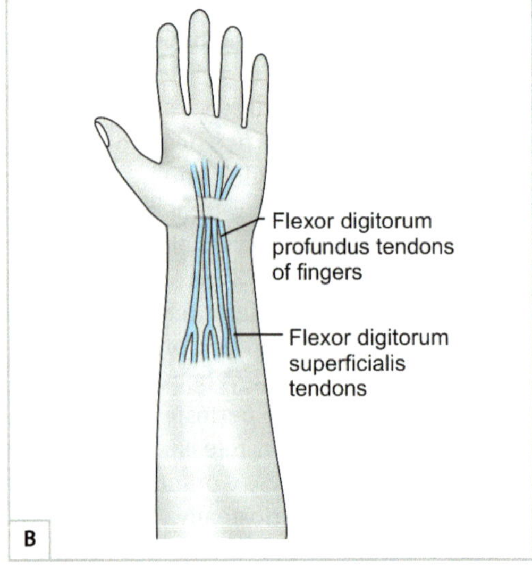

Figs 15.61.4A and B Technique of FDS to FDP transfer

is gently pulled with an artery forceps till the finger lies in the normal cascade position: metacarpophalangeal (MCP)—10°, proximal interphalangeal (PIP)—70° and distal interphalangeal (DIP)—20°. This is the attitude of the fingers in complete relaxation.
- Pull the cut end of the FDS tendon. It should glide freely forward and backward. If it does not do so, further mobilization should be done until it does so. Pull the tendon to the maximum. Make a mark on the tendon at the point, where it just becomes visible in the wound. Mark this point as "A". Now, relax the tendon and it will glide back into the forearm for a certain distance. Now, mark the point where the tendon just becomes visible at the edge of the wound. Mark this point as "B". So, the distance AB is the amplitude of movement of the FDS tendon. Mark the midpoint of the distance AB and mark this point as "C". Hold the tendon in such a way that the point "C" is just visible at the edge of the wound. This should be the position of the FDS while it is being sutured to the distal cut end of the FDP tendon.
- Pull the free end of the FDP tendon, so that the finger is held in a position of the cascade of the finger. Mark a point "D" on this tendon which corresponds to the point "C" at this position of the finger. The point "D" of the FDP must now be sutured to the FDS tendon at the point "C".
- Trim the excess length of the FDP tendon and the FDS tendons. Suturing is done with 3.0 polypropylene using modified Kessler-Mason-Allen suture.
- The procedure is repeated for the middle, ring and little fingers also.

- The tourniquet must be released and gentle pressure with a saline pad should be applied and the hand kept elevated for two minutes. Next the hand must be placed on the table and hemostasis achieved. Skin suturing is done with 3.0 ethilon and drainage tubes kept in the proximal portion of the suture line. Sterile dressings are applied and dorsal POP slab is applied with wrist in neutral position and fingers in position appropriate with the surgical procedure that has been done (nerve or tendon surgery).

Postoperative Protocol

- Admission in the ward.
- The affected hand should be kept elevated.
- Patient can take normal diet after complete recovery if he was under general anesthesia.
- Discharge of the patient by the 3rd day.
- Inspection of the suture line on the 2nd day. If necessary, a short general anesthesia may be required if the child is very serious. Suture removal can be done on the 10th day. The POP slab needs to be retained for another two weeks.
- After further two weeks, the POP is removed. The following are advised:
  - Refer to physiotherapy for active mobilization of the fingers.
  - Daily wash with soap and water.
  - Massage of scar and grafted skin with coconut oil.
  - Patient is encouraged to continue the active mobilization of the fingers for three weeks from removal of the POP.
  - After three weeks from removal of the POP, gentle passive stretching is started.

Tendon Transfer—Brachioradialis to FPL and ECRL to FDP

In a condition, where the muscles on the extensor side are acting well, these extensors can be used to provide flexion of the fingers and thumb.

Surgical Steps

- *Incision to harvest brachioradialis (BR) and FPL:* These muscles can be harvested through the exploratory incisions.

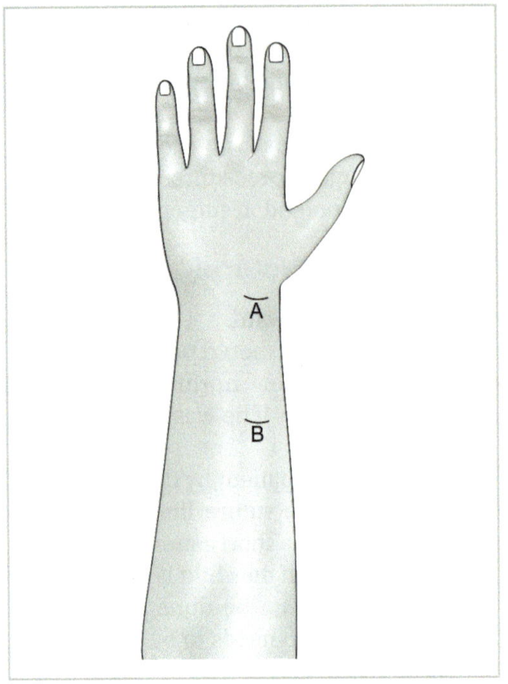

Fig. 15.61.5 Marking for the incisions for harvesting ECRL tendon

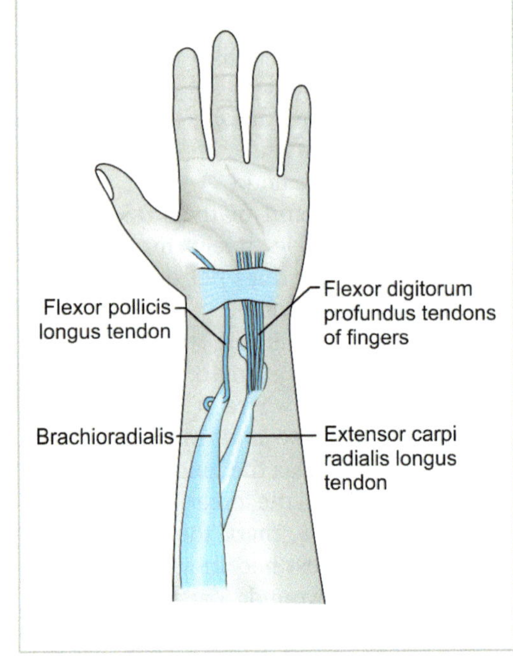

Fig. 15.61.6 After tendon suturing

- Incision for extensor carpi radialis longus (ECRL) must be made as follows (Fig. 15.61.5):
  - Incision "A" is now made. The ECRL tendon must be identified. The extensor pollicis longus (EPL) tendon runs obliquely across it and the extensor carpi radialis brevis (ECRB) tendon is on the ulnar side. The ECRL tendon should be held with a hemostat and divided closely to the insertion with a No. 11 blade.
  - Gentle traction to the ECRL is applied in a distal direction by pulling on the hemostat. This will confirm the position of the muscle proximally and the incision "B" is made now. The muscle/musculotendinous unit of the ECRL is exposed in this incision and confirmed by traction on the hemostat.
  - The FDP tendons for all the fingers are divided as proximally as possible and tagged.

Tension adjustment: The tendons of the BR must be sutured to the FPL tendon with the wrist in neutral position, thumb kept in a position of palmar abduction and interphalangeal (IP) joint in 10° flexion (Fig. 15.61.6).

- The tendon of the ECRL is sutured to the tendons of all the FDP tendons of the fingers, keeping the wrist in neutral position and fingers in a position of natural cascade: MCP—10°, PIP—70° and DIP—20°. The technique of suturing the tendons is described in the previous chapter.
- The tourniquet must be released and gentle pressure with a saline pad should be applied and the hand kept elevated for two minutes. Next, the hand must be placed on the table and hemostasis achieved. Skin suturing is done with 3.0 ethilon and drainage tubes kept in the proximal portion of the suture line. Sterile dressings are applied and dorsal POP slab is applied with wrist in neutral position and fingers

in position appropriate with the surgical procedure that has been done (nerve or tendon surgery).

Postoperative Protocol

- Admission in the ward.
- The affected hand should be kept elevated.
- Patient can take normal diet after complete recovery if he was under general anesthesia.
- Discharge of the patient by the 3rd day.
- Inspection of the suture line on the 2nd day. If necessary, a short general anesthesia may be required if the child is very serious. Suture removal can be done on the 10th day. The POP slab needs to be retained for another two weeks.
- After further two weeks, the POP is removed. The following are advised:
  - Refer to physiotherapy for active mobilization of the fingers.
  - Daily wash with soap and water.
  - Massage of scar and grafted skin with coconut oil.
  - Patient is encouraged to continue the active mobilization of the fingers for three weeks from removal of the POP.
  - After three weeks from removal of the POP, gentle passive stretching is started.

Vascularized Gracilis Muscle Transfer

62

Introduction

The transfer of the functioning gracilis muscle is the only answer to situations like some cases of brachial plexus injuries and Volkmann's ischemic contracture. The indications for such a muscle transfer have already been discussed in the previous chapters.

Advantages

- This is an easy muscle to harvest and has a pedicle of length even up to 6 to 7 cm.
- The donor site morbidity is minimal.
- It may even be possible to split the muscle for different functions like for motorizing the thumb and fingers, due to the unique anatomy of the gracilis muscle. This muscle has a dual nerve supply and the muscle fibers can be split according to the nerve fascicles supplying it.
- The muscle has a length almost equal to the length of the arm (when using the muscle as elbow flexor), and also equal to the length of the forearm (when using the muscle as finger flexor or extensor).
- The cross section of the muscle is such that it appears physiological when contracting and does not appear grotesque.
- There is no motor deficit in the lower limb after removal of the gracilis muscle.

Disadvantage

The skin paddle of this flap is not very reliable.

Surgical Steps

Donor Site Dissection

- The preferred anesthesia is either general anesthesia or combined regional block—continuous epidural anesthesia with supraclavicular block (if the surgery is for finger or hand motorization).
- Prepare for the procedure as outlined in the Appendix II.
  - Prepare the involved upper limb, including the shoulder, neck and front of chest.
  - Prepare the opposite side thigh and groin regions.

Markings (Fig. 15.62.1)

- Flex the hip to 90° and the knee to 90°. Now abduct the hip to the maximum possible. On the medial side of the thigh, the prominence of the adductor longus muscle can be seen from the pubic tubercle. Immediately posterior/inferior to this prominence, there is a small groove and within this groove is the gracilis muscle. Sometimes, it may be obvious as a small prominence in the depth of the groove;

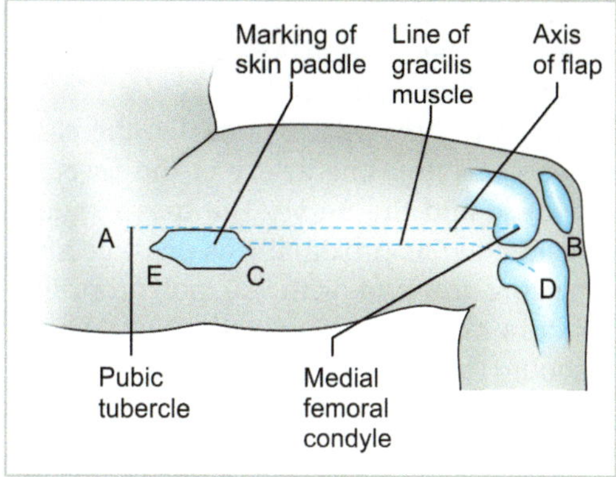

Fig. 15.62.1 Markings for the harvest of gracilis muscle

sometimes it may only be palpable in the groove. Now, mark a point on the pubic tubercle "A" and another point on the medial femoral condyle "B". Join these two lines. This forms the superior border of the gracilis muscle. It does not represent the axis of the flap. The muscle is about 2 cm inferior or behind this axis. The skin paddle can be marked now. At the proximal end of the axis, an ellipsoid skin paddle can be marked "E" about 5 cm distal to the pubic tubercle with its superior surface on the marked line. Hence, the skin paddle will lie over the muscle. The maximum size of the skin paddle can be 5 cm/8 cm.

- Mark the incision about 2 cm parallel to and inferior to the line AB. This line will start proximally at the distal tip "C" of the skin paddle and end at a point "D" on the medial side of the knee, posterior to the medial femoral condyle.
- Make the incision CD. First make the middle third of this incision. Go through the skin, superficial fascia and the deep fascia. By applying retractors on both sides of the wound, the gracilis muscle can be seen surrounded by loose areolar tissue. The adductor longus muscle can be seen superiorly and the adductor magnus inferiorly.
- The gracilis muscle can be dissected free from the loose areolar tissue. There will be a few minor vascular pedicles entering the muscle belly. These can be divided and ligated.
- On the proximal third, the incision can be made on the proximal part of the line CD up to the point "C". From here, the incision will continue on the superior border of the skin paddle. When the incision is deepened through the deep fascia, anchoring sutures must be made between the deep fascia and the skin paddle to prevent shearing of the myocutaneous perforator. Only the skin flap on the superior edge of the incision should be raised now.
- The adductor longus muscle will come into view (Fig. 15.62.2). A retractor must be placed and the adductor longus muscle retracted superiorly, to expose the undersurface of this muscle. Now, the vascular pedicle can be seen entering the undersurface of the gracilis muscle. There will be one or two branches from the pedicle to the adductor longus muscle that should be carefully ligated and cut. Similarly, the branches to the adductor magnus muscle can also be ligated and divided. This will allow further retraction of the adductor longus muscle and further expose the vascular pedicle.
- About 3 cm proximal to the vascular hilum, the nerve can be seen and dissected. This is the anterior branch of the obturator nerve. This must be gently dissected proximally as the nerve lies on the surface of the adductor magnus muscle. The greater the length of the nerve that is dissected, the easier is the nerve anastomosis at the recipient site.
- When the entry point of the vascular pedicle is made out on the medial/undersurface of the gracilis muscle, the incision on the inferior edge of the skin paddle can be made. Anchoring sutures should be placed again between the deep fascia and the dermis of the skin paddle. Now, the dissection should go on the undersurface of the gracilis muscle and any branches to the adductor magnus muscle should be ligated and divided. This

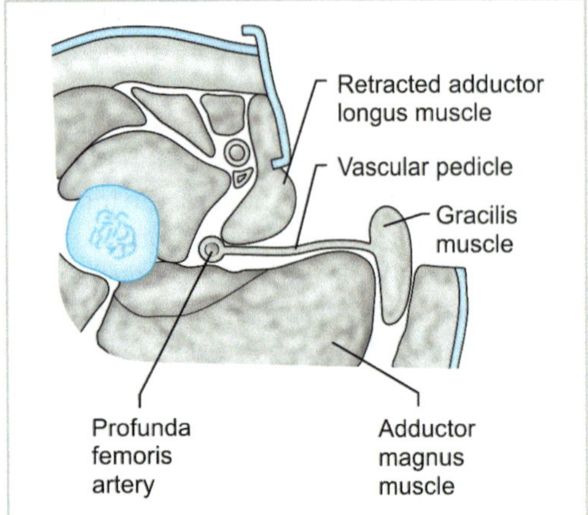

Fig. 15.62.2 Dissection of the vascular pedicle

will totally free the circumference of the muscle, which will now be attached by the vascular pedicle and the nerve only.

- Identify the origin of the gracilis muscle from the pubic tubercle and dissect it.
- Now, complete the distal third of the incision. Go through the superficial and deep fascia. The muscle can be followed up to its insertion on the medial femoral condyle as a thin tendon. This tendon will lie between the sartorius superiorly and the semitendinosus inferiorly.
- Mark every 5 cm on the muscle with a 3.0 silk suture. This step is to ensure that when the muscle is transplanted, the optimal length will be maintained and will neither be lengthened nor shortened.
- Now, divide the origin of the gracilis muscle, as close to the pubic tubercle as possible. This may be tendinous at some areas. The division of the origin can be done using cautery.
- Divide the tendinous insertion.
- Observe the bleeding from the edges of the skin paddle. Make a streak on the surface of the skin paddle with a needle tip and note the nature of the bleed. This will serve as a monitoring skin flap in the postoperative period.
- Now, the muscle lies free, attached only by the vascular pedicle and the nerve. These should be divided only after the recipient site has been prepared to shorten the warm ischemia time.
- *Division of the pedicle:* Usually, there are two veins and one artery at the vascular pedicle and the nerve. The nerve should be divided as proximally as possible after tagging the end with 7.0 polypropylene suture materials as a marker. Soft clamps should be applied over the artery and veins. The proximal ends of the artery and veins should be ligated with 3.0 vicryl. The vessels should be divided and the time noted. The flap should be placed on a moist abdominal pad and taken to the recipient site for vascular anastomosis.
- *Management of the donor site:* After securing hemostasis, the secondary defect should be closed in layers with subcutaneous suturing with 3.0 vicryl and the skin closed primarily with 3.0 ethilon after keeping a suction drain. Sterile dressings should be applied and elastocrépe bandage applied over it.

Vascular Anastomosis

- The flap is brought to the hand defect. First, the flap is held up and the pedicle allowed to hang down. This step will make sure that there is no inadvertent twisting of the vascular pedicle. The flap is then placed over the defect with the correct orientation and the end of the pedicle should be placed over the recipient vessels. A few sutures should be applied to inset the flap.
- The recipient vessels should be divided, blood flow checked from the divided artery and approximator clamps applied. The soft clamps must be released from the donor vessels. Vascular anastomosis should be done (The technique of vascular anastomosis is beyond the scope of this manual).

Recipient Site Dissection

It depends on whether the gracilis is being used to bring about (I) elbow flexion or (II) finger flexion (Table 15.62.1).

Table 15.62.1	Recipient site dissection of vascularized gracilis muscle transfer	
	Transfer I	***Transfer II***
Aim	To bring about elbow flexion and finger extension	To bring about finger flexion
New origin	Lateral aspect of clavicle and acromion process	II, III and IV ribs
New insertion	Into the finger extensors with the brachioradialis as pulley	Into the finger flexors and flexor pollicis longus (FPL) tendon
Donor vessels	Thoracoacromial vessels/or transverse cervical vessels	Thoracodorsal vessels
Donor nerves	Spinal accessory nerve/contralateral C7/intercostal nerves 3–6	Intercostal nerves 3–6

SECTION

16

Difficult Hand Problems

The Mutilated Hand

63

Introduction

Mutilated hands are those in which there has been a loss of composite tissues which may be either skin, soft tissues, bones, tendons or fingers themselves. Thus, mutilated hands result in disability of varying degrees. A minimum of three structures should be lost before it can be called a mutilated hand.

Mutilated hands can present in the emergency situation or can present in the outpatient clinic after many attempts have been made at reconstruction. When such patients present to surgeons, it is very essential to do what is best for him, as the disability with which the patient presents may be extreme.

To simplify the method of assessing the defect, hand mutilations can be classified as follows:

Surface Mutilation

- Dorsal
- Palmar
- Ulnar
- Radial.

The basic work-up of such patients is threefold:

- Assess what is lost. (THE DEFECT)
- How to reconstruct the defect? (THE PLAN)
- When to carry out the plan? (THE TIMING)

Terminal Mutilation

The basic requirements for a functioning hand are the following:

- *Ulnar post:* Consisting of a minimum of two fingers.
- *Radial post:* Consisting of a thumb.
- *Thumb web:* The connecting structure between the radial post and the ulnar post.

Radial Post

Though, it quantifies that there must be at least two fingers, there are also some qualifying criteria:

- The fingers that are available must have a critical length up to the middle of the middle phalanx (MPX) of the finger.
- The metacarpophalangeal (MCP) joints of the available fingers must be mobile.
- They must have sensate tips.
- The two fingers that are available can be:
  - The index and middle fingers: In which case the power grips of the hand may not be effective?
  - The middle and ring fingers: In which most of the function in the hand can be achieved?
  - The ring and little fingers: In which case, not only precision grips on the hand are impaired, but the total power of the hand is also impaired, because the motors of the little finger are not powerful enough.
  - Hence, if no fingers are available and reconstruction is planned, it would be ideal to reconstruct middle and ring fingers.

Ulnar Post Absent

Surgical option and level of amputation of ulnar post is described in Table 16.63.1.

Radial post: This is represented by the thumb. The thumb must be of critical length, up to the neck of the proximal phalanx. If this length is not available, the thumb must be reconstructed up to this level at least.

Radial Post Absent

Surgical option, characteristics, level of amputation of radial post is described in Table 16.63.2.

Thumb Web Absent

Surgical option and characteristic of thumb web is described in Table 16.63.3.

Table 16.63.1 Surgical option and level of amputation of ulnar post

Level of amputation				*Surgical option*
Index	*Middle*	*Ring*	*Little*	
–	+	+	+	Ray amputation of index finger
–	–	+	+	No surgery required: There will be some loss of power
–	–	–	+	Augment with double toe transfer
–	–	–	–	Augment with double toe transfer—middle and ring fingers
+	–	–	–	Augment with double toe transfer
+	+	–	–	No surgery required: There will be some loss of power
+	+	+	–	Ray amputation of little finger
+	–	+	–	Shift index finger ray to middle finger ray
–	+	–	+	Shift little finger ray to ring finger ray

Table 16.63.2 Surgical option, characteristics and level of amputation of radial post

Level of amputation	*Characteristic*	*Surgical option*
Amputation proximal to the neck of the proximal phalanx, up to the metacarpophalangeal joint	• Patient not willing for toe transfer • Not willing for microsurgery • Expertise not available for microsurgery	Osteoplastic reconstruction
		Vascularized wrap around great toe transfer
	In children	Vascularized second toe transfer
Amputation proximal to the metacarpophalangeal joint to the base of the metacarpal bone with intact carpometacarpal joint	Expertise not available for microsurgery	Pollicization and opponensplasty
	Microsurgical expertise available	Vascularized second toe transfer and opponensplasty
Amputation through the carpometacarpal joint with destroyed joint	Expertise not available for microsurgery	Pollicization
	Microsurgical expertise available	Vascularized transmetatarsal second toe transfer

Table 16.63.3 Surgical option and characteristic of thumb web

Thumb web not present	Characteristic	Surgical option
	Contracted thumb web—moderate	Release by: • Z plasty • Square flap
	Contracted thumb web—severe	Release and flap cover: • Groin flap • Posterior interosseous artery flap

Sequence of Surgery

When all three components: (1) the radial post, (2) the ulnar post and (3) the thumb web are not available, reconstruction of all the three components is prescribed as discussed above.

- First the ulnar post must be reconstructed.
- Next the thumb web must be reconstructed.
- Finally, the thumb must be reconstructed.

There must be a minimum period of three months between two procedures.

Prosthetics

Training Prosthesis

When the patient presents with a loss of fingers or thumb, the remaining digits usually lose their useful function because they have nothing to act against. For example, when the fingers are not present, the thumb loses its capacity to pronate. This will lead to a functionless hand even after the reconstruction of the fingers, because the thumb is not useful. To make such thumbs to be trained, it is advisable to attach a prosthesis to the ulnar post that the thumb can act against.

Functional Prosthesis

These are usually prescribed for more proximal amputations, to achieve basic function.

Cosmetic Prosthesis

Cosmetic prosthesis can be prescribed for loss of tips of fingers.

Vascularized Double Toe Transfer

64

Indications

A double toe transfer of the contralateral second and third toes on a single pedicle is indicated for loss of contiguous fingers of the hand. Typically, the stumps must be at the level of the metacarpal heads, so that the metacarpophalangeal joints can be reconstructed.

If the amputation of the fingers is more proximal, i.e. at the level of mid-metacarpals, it is ideal to augment the stump with a nonvascularized bone graft and skin flap, before the double toe transfer is done. This is because, the double toe harvest should only be done at the level of the metatarsophalangeal joints of the second and third toes. If the toes are cut proximally, the stability of the foot will be lost.

Preparation

- Palpate the dorsalis pedis artery and mark the course on the opposite foot.
- Put the leg in a dependent position and mark the main dorsal veins, the transverse arch and the great saphenous system.
- Mark a dorsal triangle on the dorsum of the foot, encircling the second and third toes (Figs 16.64.1A and B). The medial limit of the base of this dorsal triangle should not cross the midpoint of the first web space between the great toe and the second toe. Similarly, the lateral limit of the dorsal triangle should not cross the midpoint of the third web space between the third and fourth toes. The apex of the triangle should be about 1.5 cm proximal to the web space between the second and third toes. Mark the plantar triangle slightly smaller than the dorsal triangle.
- Mark a point "A" at the level of the distal edge of the inferior extensor retinaculum, halfway between the dorsalis pedis artery marking and the great saphenous system marking.
- Draw a curvilinear line between the point "A" and the apex of the marked triangle.
- Similarly, from the apex of the triangle on the plantar aspect, make a marking that extends from the apex proximally along the second metatarsal to the midsole.

Surgical Steps

- Prepare the ipsilateral lower limb from the knee distally and apply the drapings.
- The tourniquet can be raised and the time noted.
- Make the dorsal incision down to the dermis only.
- Raise medial and lateral flaps for about 2 to 3 cm on either side.
- The following should be dissected now—the great saphenous vein, other dorsal veins, fat and subcutaneous tissue.

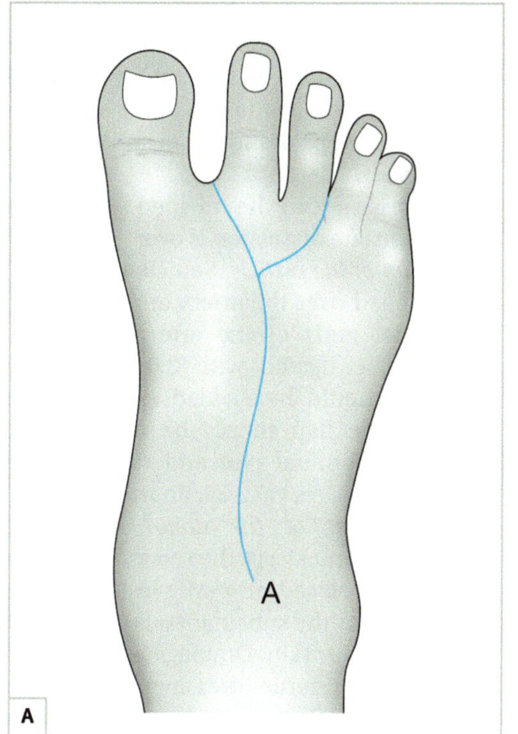

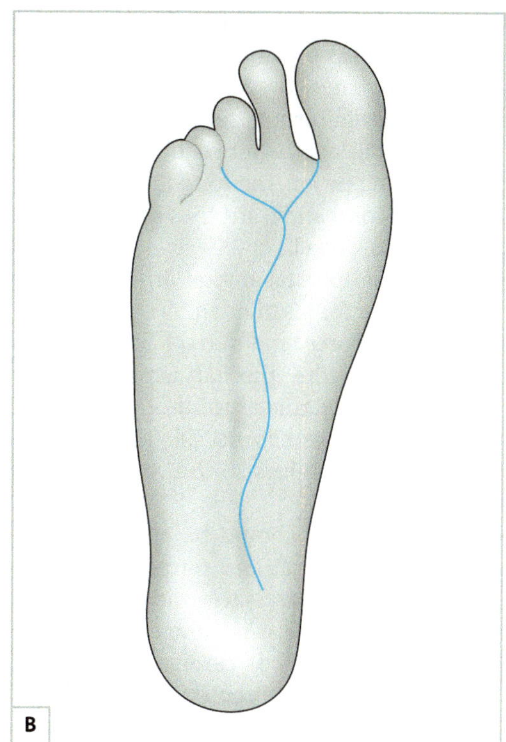

Figs 16.64.1A and B Markings for the double toe transfer

- Dissect the dorsalis pedis artery up to the distal part of the intermetatarsal space, where it will divide into two branches to the great toe and the second toe.
- Dissect the deep peroneal nerve which lies deep to the dorsalis pedis artery. Dissect it till the divisions to the great toe and the second toe. Tease gently and separate the fascicles to the great toe and second toe. Divide the fascicles to the second toe as proximally as possible and tag with 7.0 polypropylene.
- Dissect the extensor hallucis longus tendon of both the second and third toes and divide it at the level of the distal edge of the inferior extensor retinaculum. Divide the tendon of the extensor brevis at the level of the metatarsal base.
- At the distal part of the dorsalis pedis artery, identify the deep communicating branch going to the plantar side. This branch will join with the first plantar metatarsal artery to form the plantar digital artery. And this plantar digital artery will divide into two: the medial plantar digital artery going to the lateral side of great toe and the lateral plantar digital artery going to the second toe. Examine this system to see which is dominant—the first dorsal metatarsal artery and the dorsal digital arteries or the first plantar metatarsal arteries and the plantar digital arteries.
- Now surgeons go to the plantar side dissection. Make the plantar incisions. The medial and lateral plantar digital nerves are identified. The fascicles to the great toe and the fascicles to the second toe teased from the second medial digital nerve. The fascicles going to the second toe are cut as proximal as possible and tagged with 7.0 polypropylenes. Similarly, the plantar digital nerve to the second and

third toes is dissected and the nerve is cut as proximal as possible and tagged with 7.0 polypropylenes.

- The flexor digitorum brevis muscle is cut at the midsole level, where it joins the tendon of the long flexor. The long flexor tendons of the second and third toes are divided at the midsole level.
- The medial plantar digital artery (branch to the great toe) is divided.
- The transverse metatarsal ligament is divided on the medial aspect of the metatarsophalangeal joint of the second toe. Great care should be taken at this level to avoid injury to the vessels at this level.
- Now, retractors should be applied to the second metatarsal and retracted laterally and the first metatarsal retracted medially. The arterial system is now exposed. The system should be carefully dissected, taking into account the dominance of the vessel system. This can be assisted by carefully dividing the interosseous muscles and further exposing the arterial system.
- Now, the second and third toes are almost completely dissected as a single unit and held only by the intact metatarsal bone and the artery and veins. The capsule of the second and third toe metatarsophalangeal joints are now incised proximally, near the attachment to the metatarsal bone. This incision should be taken on the volar aspect and both joints disarticulated from their respective metatarsals. Thus, a cuff of capsule and volar plate should be harvested along with the two toes.
- Once the disarticulation is over, the remaining soft tissues can be divided. This includes the third plantar artery system, so that the double toe flap is now held only by the arteries and veins.
- Now release the tourniquet, apply warm, moist pads over the double toes and the vascular pedicle. Take care to prevent the toe from falling down and shearing the vessels. Raise the foot for about 5 minutes. Then place the foot on the table. It usually takes about 15 to 20 minutes for the circulation to be re-established in the dissected toes. By the end of this time, the toes become pink and warm and ready for transfer.
- The vessels can be divided when the recipient site dissection is over.
- *Division of the pedicle:* Soft clamps should be applied over the artery and veins. The proximal ends of the artery and veins should be ligated with 3.0 vicryl. The vessels should be divided and the time noted. The flap should be placed on a moist abdominal pad and taken to the recipient site for vascular anastomosis.
- *Management of the donor site:* After securing hemostasis, the secondary defect should be closed primarily in layers with 3.0 vicryl for the subcutaneous tissues and 4.0 ethilon for skin. Drainage tubes should be placed. Sterile dressings should be applied and elastocrépe bandage applied over it. A posterior below knee plaster of Paris (POP) slab should be applied.

Recipient Site Dissection

- The hand is prepared as described in Appendix I and Appendix II.
- A curvilinear incision is made over the anatomical snuff box area and the following structures are identified and dissected:
  - The radial artery and both venae comitantes
  - The cephalic vein
  - The superficial branch of the radial nerve.
- One percent of xylocaine gauze is applied over the dissected vessels.
- A volar incision is made on the palm of the hand proximal to the stumps of the middle and ring fingers. Raise the medial and lateral skin flaps, apply anchoring sutures

with 3.0 ethilon and dissect the following structures:
- The flexor digitorum profundus tendons of the middle and ring fingers.
- The digital nerves to the middle and ring fingers—the ends should be tagged with 7.0 polypropylenes.

- Similarly, make an incision on the dorsum of the hand proximal to the stumps of the middle and ring fingers. Dissect the following structures and keep ready:
  - The extensor digitorum tendons of the middle and ring fingers.
  - Prepare the heads of the metacarpals of the middle and ring fingers, to which double toe flap is going to be attached.
- Apply gentle compression with moist gauze and padding over the wound. Release the tourniquet. Hold the hand in an elevated position for a period of 4 to 5 minutes. Rest the hand on the table and secure hemostasis.

Fixation of the Double Toe Flap

- Bring the double toe flap to the recipient site. Place the toes over the stumps of the middle and ring fingers and get a good position, a position in which good opposition can be achieved with the fingers and is a functional position.
- A subcutaneous tunnel is created between the recipient site vessels and the summit of the stump. This tunnel is for the vessels of the double toe flap to be passed through to reach the recipient vessels—the radial artery.
- The structures to be passed through the tunnel are:
  - The arteries
  - The veins
  - The deep peroneal nerve.
- *Fixation:* It is done by repairing the joint capsule of the second and third toes with the joint capsules/soft tissues around the heads of the middle and ring fingers respectively. The reconstruction of the joint capsules is done with 4.0 polypropylenes.
- If the toes still appear unstable, they can be stabilized with short oblique K-wires without causing damage to the vessels.
- *Tendon repair:* The flexor longus tendons of the toes are sutured to the flexor digitorum profundus tendons of the middle and ring fingers, and the extensor longus tendons of the toes are sutured to the ends of the extensor digitorum tendons of the middle and ring fingers. The tension should be adjusted, so that, the toes are stable and in a functional position. The repair is done with 3.0 polypropylenes using modified Kessler-Mason-Allen suture technique.
- *Nerve repair:* The digital nerves are sutured to the two plantar digital nerves of the toes and the deep peroneal nerve is sutured to the superficial branch of the radial nerve at the anatomical snuff box. The nerve repairs are done with 7.0 polypropylenes using epineural sutures.
- *Vascular anastomosis*: The recipient vessels should be divided, blood flow checked from the divided artery and approximator clamps applied. The soft clamps must be released from the donor vessels. Vascular anastomosis should be done (The technique of vascular anastomosis is beyond the scope of this manual).

SECTION 17

Appendices

Preparation for Hand Surgery

I

Introduction

When the patient is put on the table for surgery, the position of the patient is important. For any standard hand surgical procedure, supine position of the patient is ideal. Even if surgery is planned on both the hands, they can be performed with the patient in the supine position.

Before the actual surgery is performed, there are certain things to be made ready.

- *Getting the electrocautery equipment ready:* Usually, only the bipolar cautery is used in hand surgical procedures. However, in procedures like the use of pedicled latissimus dorsi muscle flap and some procedures on the upper arm, monopolar cautery may be used. Hence, these equipments must be made ready.
- *Getting the tourniquet ready:* The recommended tourniquet for use in hand surgery is the pneumatic tourniquet, where the calibration of the pressure used is clear. The tourniquet cuff must be applied at the level of the upper arm of the side that is going to be operated.
- *Applying the monitors:* Like the pulse oximeter and noninvasive blood pressure (BP) monitors.
- *Setting up the intravenous line:* Called traditionally the "life-line", this IV line will serve as a portal for drug delivery and for resuscitation if there is a fall in the general condition of the patient.
- *Catheterizing the urinary bladder:* This is particularly important when the surgery may take a long time, or if the condition of the patient must be monitored closely.
- *Giving the prophylactic antibiotic:* A dose of antibiotic is given as soon as the patient is put on the table. This is followed up with one dose after 12 hours and the next after another 12 hours.
- *Checking required materials for the procedure:* Like the silastic rods or silastic materials which may be needed in cases like staged tendon reconstruction, external fixators and autoclaved set of plates and screws along with AO instruments which may be needed in bone surgery on the hand.
- *Getting drugs ready for use during the surgical procedure*: Some drugs may be required to be given during the course of the procedure. For example, during a replantation procedure, a bolus dose of injection heparin may be required to be given intravenously just before release of clamps. Hence, it is important to have the required drugs ready for use.
- *Wearing the surgical loupe:* The basic requirements for a good hand surgery are:
  - Good lighting
  - Good anesthesia
  - Good tourniquet

- Good magnification
- Good technique.

Hence, it is important for the surgeon and the surgical assistant to wear surgical loupes. Magnification makes identifying structures easier, avoids excessive force on delicate tissues and ultimately benefits the patient.

Preparation and Draping of the Hand

- The upper limb is prepared from the elbow downward in any hand procedure.
- *Draping:* Two towels on the hand table, one towel to cover the arm with the tourniquet, and one sheet to cover the patient.

Preparation for a Free Flap

II

Preparation Before the Patient is Brought to the Operation Theater

Before the patient is brought to the operation theater, the following should already have been done. These should not be done on the table or after anesthesia has been given.

- *Doppler:* A Doppler study to analyze the vascular pattern in the patient and an appropriate plan must be ready.
- *Markings:* When the Doppler study has been done, the appropriate markings for the flap should be made preoperatively and the plan explained to the patient immediately. Any alternate plan if made should also be informed to the patient and consent obtained for the same.
- *Lint:* Once the marking for the flap has been made, a lint pattern must be cut, given to the operating room personnel for autoclaving and to be kept ready for use during surgery.
- *Measurements:* The accurate measurements must be made before the patient is wheeled into the operating room. For example, the length of the second toe required for a toe transfer must be made preoperatively, with the help of relevant X-rays of the foot, the opposite hand for an X-ray of the normal thumb, etc.
- *Photographs:* Clinical photographs are a must. But, they must be taken preoperatively, with appropriate positioning of the patient. Sometimes, movement videos may be required, which may not be possible if the patient has been anesthetized.

Only after the above conditions have been fulfilled, the patient may be put on the operating table. Once the patient is on the table, he is under the care of an anesthesiologist, who should be given freedom of space and time to decide on the anesthesia.

Preparation While Anesthesia is Being Delivered

While anesthesia is being delivered, the following should be arranged:

- *Microsurgery chart:* This is a form that records the main events of the microsurgical procedure. A sample of this form is shown in the section on proformas. It is the duty of the surgeon to allocate the duty of filling out this form to a responsible person.
- *Instruments:* The microinstruments that are required, any special instruments that may be required, should be arranged on a tray.

Preparation After the Anesthesia has been Delivered

- *Positioning of patient:* Once the anesthesia has been given, the patient can be put into position for surgery. This may be determined by the procedure that is being done, or the number of teams that are going to operate.

- *Tourniquets to be applied:* Tourniquets should be applied at the appropriate parts.
- *Setting up of the various equipment*: Before the surgeon can go to wash up, the following equipment must be positioned in such a way that it is convenient for the surgeon, convenient for monitoring of the patient by the anesthetist, convenient for the staff nurses and the paramedical personnel to carry out their duties.
  - Microscope
  - Bipolar and unipolar cautery machine
  - Patient vitals monitoring machine
  - Tourniquet machines
  - Compressed air sources
  - Video monitor from the microscope.
- *Earthpad for cautery*: Appropriate placement of the earthpad for cautery should be done now, after the position of the patient has been determined.
- *Bladder catheterization:* The next step to be done is catheterization of the bladder. This step is very important for monitoring of the patient, especially in this surgery which may be prolonged. When this has been done, the surgeon can wash up.
- *Preparation and draping*: Now, the preparation and draping of the patient can be done. Only after the draping, the following can be procured and placed in the surgical field.
  - Bipolar cautery leads and wires
  - Unipolar cautery leads and wires
- *Start of surgery*: Now the surgery can be started. Apart from all the above, one more thing is very important, especially when a microsurgery procedure is being done. This is decorum in the theater.

Preparing Instrument Sets for Use in Hand Surgery

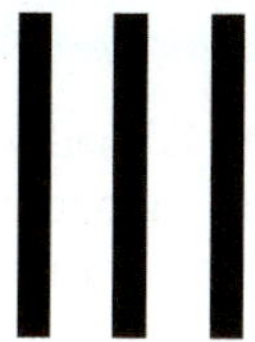

Preparing Instrument Sets

Following are the preparing instrument sets for use in hand surgery:

- Axillary block pack
- Basic set
- Tendon set
- Bone set

Axillary Block Set

It consists of the following:

- One sheet
- One kidney tray
- 20 ml glass syringe
- 1 IV needle (20 g)
- 2 IM needles (24 g)
- One sponge holder
- One stainless steel cup
- One towel

Basic Set

It consists of the following:

- Two sheets
- Two towels
- Two aprons
- 5 ml syringe
- 1 IV needle (20 g)
- 1 IM needle (24 g)
- 6" fine dissecting scissors—one pair
- Toothed forceps—one pair
- Nontoothed forceps—one pair
- Mosquito-curved artery forceps—two pairs
- Mosquito-straight artery forceps—two pairs
- one pair—skin hooks
- one pair—cats paw retractors
- One needle holder—7"
- One sponge holding forceps
- One kidney tray
- One stainless steel cup
- One towel clip
- One blood pressure (BP) handle

Bone Set

Bone set consists of the following:

- Bone nibbler
- Bone cutter
- Autoclavable hand drill with chuck
- K-wires set
- Wire cutter
- Periosteal elevator
- Gigli saw
- Chisel
- Osteotome
- Mallet
- Self-retaining retractor

Skin Graft Set

Skin graft set consists of the following:

- One sheet
- One stainless steel tray
- Two Gamgee pads (size 15 cm × 10 cm)
- 10 bandage rolls
- Skin graft handle
- Two wooden retractors (wooden plates).

Microsurgery Instruments Tray

This is used only for microsurgical procedures and hence requires careful handling and storage. This tray should not be autoclaved and is sterilized by formalin tablets. It contains the following instruments.

- Fine dissecting scissors—straight
- Fine dissecting scissors—curved
- Micro scissors—straight
- Micro scissors—curved
- Micro forceps—two pairs
- Micro-needle holder
- Vessel dilator
- Soft clamps—four numbers.
- Approximator clamps—two numbers
- Background material
- Metal scale.

Harvesting a Sural Nerve Graft

IV

The sural nerve graft is quite commonly used in hand surgery in the following situations:

- In brachial plexus injuries where nerve gaps have to be reconstructed.
- Conditions where loss of nerve occurs following trauma or tumors.

Surgical Steps

- First prepare and drape the entire leg and foot from which the nerve is to be harvested.
- Mark the course of the nerve:
  - Mark the lateral malleolus and the lateral border of the tendo-achilles at the level of the lateral malleolus. Mark the midpoint "A" of the distance between the lateral malleolus and the lateral border of the tendo-achilles.
  - Now consider the calf region of the leg and note the level of maximum convexity of this region. Mark the midpoint "B" of the maximal convexity on the calf region (Fig. 17.IV.1).

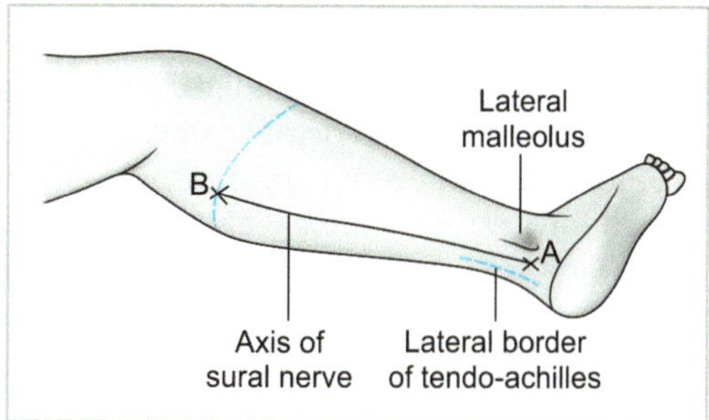

Fig. 17.IV.1 Markings for harvesting a sural nerve graft

  - Draw the line AB. This marks the course of the sural nerve.
- The surgery can be done under local anesthetic infiltration.
- The incision is made over the point "A" and extended proximally for about 5 cm along the marked line AB, through the skin and subcutaneous tissues.
- The skin edges are retracted and the sural nerve is dissected. It runs alongside the lesser saphenous vein and this vein should not be mistaken for the nerve.
- A skin hook is applied on the nerve and lifted up. Gentle traction is applied to make the nerve taut. The proximal course of the taut nerve can be palpated under the skin along the marked line AB. The skin incision is extended further proximally for another 5 cm and the nerve is dissected.
- This step is repeatedly done with the help of retraction of the skin hook, till the point "B", with where the nerve may be embedded in the superficial layers of the gastrocnemius muscle.
- Once the dissection of the nerve is complete, an identification stitch is made with 7.0 polypropylenes on the end of the nerve at the calf region. This is because the nerve should be reversed when it is used as a graft and the identification stitch will identify the distal end.
- Both ends of the dissected nerve are divided with no. 11 blade to ensure a clean cut.
- The harvested nerve graft is stored in cup of normal saline till it is used.

Harvesting a Skin Graft

V

A skin graft is required in many of the reconstructive procedures in hand surgery. It is therefore essential that the hand surgeon be adept in taking skin grafts of varying thickness according to the situation.

The materials required for harvesting a skin graft can be prepared in the form of a packed set that can be used when required. The preparation of this skin graft set has been outlined in the Appendix on preparation of sets for surgery.

The requirement of skin graft is of two categories in hand surgery:

- The first type is the small graft required for a part of a single finger alone. An example would be the donor site of a cross finger flap. This small skin graft can be harvested from the medial side of the upper arm. The advantage of harvesting a small graft in this site is that it is done in the same field of anesthesia (axillary block), it is not cosmetically disfiguring as it is hidden and it does not require many dressings in the form of Gamgee pads and bandages as would be required for a dressing on the thigh.
- The second type is the requirement of a large sheet or sheets of skin graft to cover extensive raw areas on the forearms or hand, or to cover the donor site of a large flap like the radial artery forearm flap or posterior interosseous flap. This will have to be harvested from the thigh/thighs.

The first type is described in the section on cross finger flap. The method of harvesting a skin graft from the thigh will be discussed here.

Surgical Steps

- This surgery requires an anesthesia of the lower limbs and this must be informed to the anesthetist at the beginning of the procedure on the hand.
- Ask a theater assistant to hold up the opposite side leg and prepare the thigh with antiseptic solution from the inguinal region to just below the knee.
- Apply two sterile sheets on the table, covering also the unprepared lower limb. Now place a sterile towel lengthwise on the sterile sheets and receive the unprepared leg. Drape this part securely and apply a sterile bandage to secure it. Then a sterile sheet can be placed over the abdomen.
- Paint the thigh again with antiseptic solution.
- Apply a disposable skin graft blade in the graft handle and adjust the thickness.
- Harvest a graft from the thigh, preferring the medial side, for cosmetic reasons.
- Place the skin graft in normal saline solution. Apply a moist abdominal pad over the area where the skin graft has been taken and apply gentle pressure. Wait for 2 minutes and then gently remove the

pad. Apply paraffin gauze over the site in a single layer to cover the entire area.

- Place gauze pieces that have been soaked in betadine solution over the paraffin gauze, to again cover the entire area. Apply Gamgee pads over the betadine gauze and the circumference of the thigh and roll sterile bandages over the entire thigh. The bandaging should be secure and should apply gentle compression. This can be enhanced by applying a crepe bandage over the dressing.

Harvesting an Ulnar Bone Graft

VI

Surgical Steps

- The upper limb is prepared up to above the elbow.
- A gentle "S"-shaped incision is marked over the subcutaneous border of the ulna just distal to the olecranon. This incision should be about 8 cm long. The incision is made deeply, down to the bone (Fig. 17.VI.1).
- The incision is made on the periosteum and the periosteum elevated on both sides to expose the ulna for a width of about 3 cm.
- The required dimensions of the bone are now marked on the ulna. The length of the bone required is the length of the thumb with 1 cm extra. The width should be 2 cm.
- Perform the osteotomy to raise the cortico cancellous bone graft. If the bone graft is going to be pegged into a single bone, the graft should be sculpted into the shape of a "cricket bat", to enable the "handle" end to be pegged into the head of the bone. If the bone graft is to be inserted between two ends of bone, as is done when doing a surgery for nonunion, the bone graft should be sculpted in the form of a "ladle" or a "roti belan", with a "handle" on either end (Figs 17.VI.2A and B).
- Place the bone graft in normal saline.
- Close the donor site of the bone graft in layers with 3.0 vicryl for the subcutaneous tissues and 4.0 ethilon for skin. Drainage tubes should be placed. Sterile dressings should be applied.

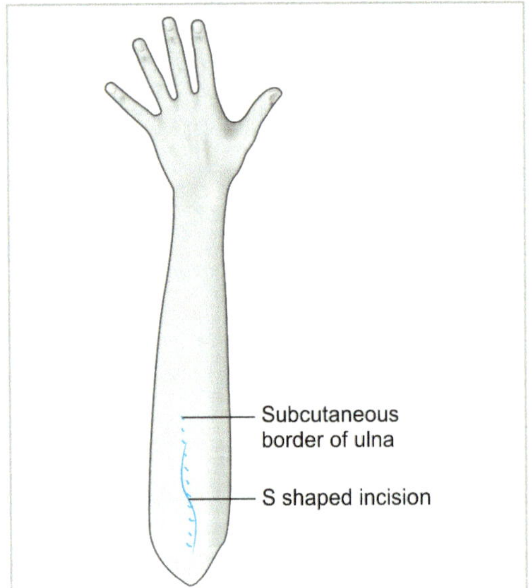

Fig. 17.VI.1 Markings for harvesting an ulnar bone graft

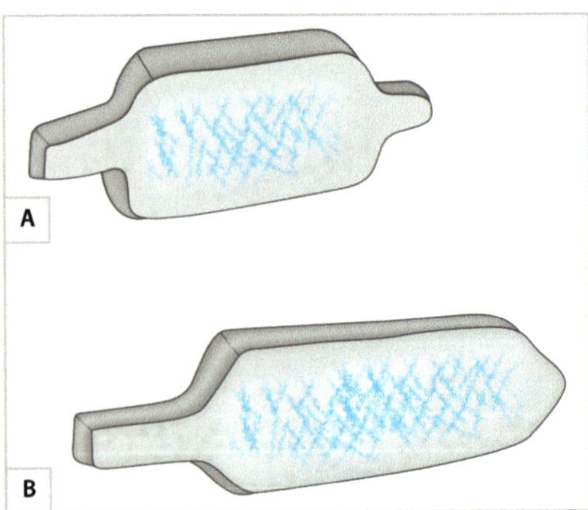

Figs 17.VI.2A and B Sculpted shapes of the ulnar bone graft

Harvesting a Palmaris Longus Tendon Graft

VII

The palmaris longus (PL) is first tested preoperatively by asking the patient to touch the tips of the thumb and little finger and then flexing the wrist. This will make two tendons prominent on the central half of the flexor aspect of the forearm near the wrist, if the PL is present. The other tendon that becomes prominent is the flexor carpi radialis tendon. However, if the PL is absent, only the flexor carpi radialis tendon will become prominent.

Surgical Steps

- The hand and forearm are prepared as described in Appendix I.
- The first incision is about 2.0 cm, made at the level of the volar wrist crease over the palpated PL tendon.
- The tendon is dissected at this level by freeing it from the numerous fibrous strands that connect it to the overlying skin and the surrounding structures. Once it is totally dissected, it is divided and a hemostat applied on the cut end.
- Another incision about 2.0 cm is made about 6 to 7 cm more proximally on the forearm after applying traction on the cut end of the tendon and palpating the taut tendon under the skin (Fig. 17.VII.1).
- The PL is retrieved through this wound, and the hemostat reapplied at the cut end.

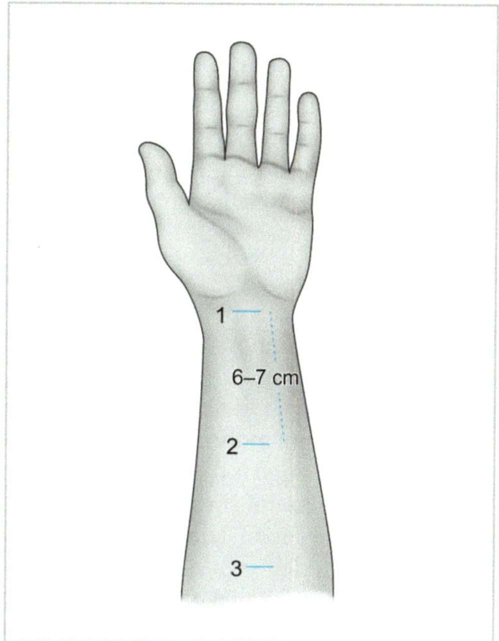

Fig. 17.VII.1 Markings for harvesting a PL tendon graft

- Again another incision is made proximal to the above incision and the PL tendon is divided close to the musculotendinous junction.
- The tendon is placed in a cup of normal saline till its use.

Harvesting a Fascia Lata Graft

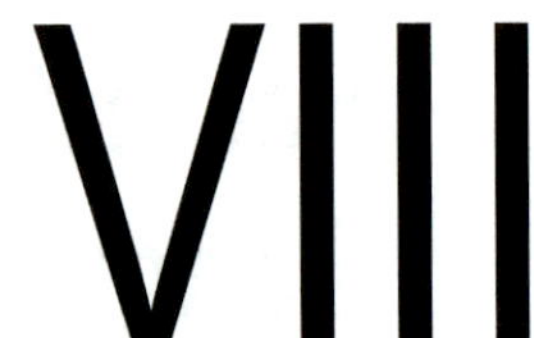

When tendon grafts are required for flexor tendon reconstruction of more than one finger or extensor tendon reconstruction of more than two fingers, the PL tendon graft will not be enough. Hence, a larger tendon graft is required. The alternate source of a tendon graft is the fascia lata graft.

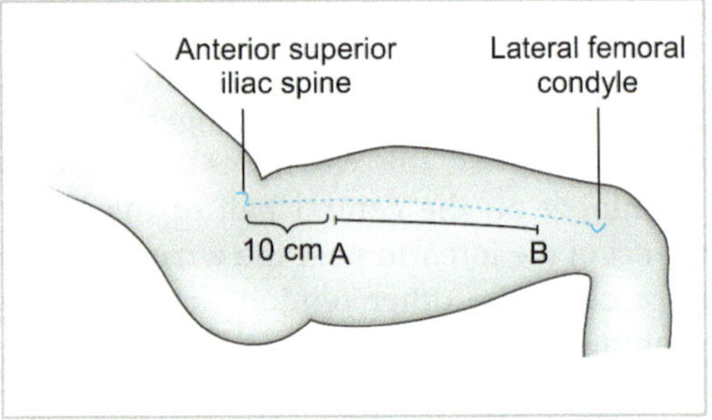

Fig. 17.VIII.1 Markings for harvesting a fascia lata graft

Surgical Steps

- This procedure can be done under local anesthetic infiltration or infiltration of tumescent solution.
- The thigh is prepared from the level of the inguinal ligament to the knee.
- *Markings:* The thigh is flexed and adducted to expose the lateral surface. This position will make the fascia lata taut. It extends from the anterior superior iliac spine to the knee. The width of the fascia is about 10 cm and the anterior limit is the imaginary line drawn from the anterior superior iliac spine to the lateral femoral condyle.
- A longitudinal incision AB is marked about 4 cm posterior to the marking of the anterior limit of the fascia lata. The length of this incision should be about 4 cm longer than the requirement of tendon graft. The proximal limit of the incision is 10 cm from the anterior superior iliac spine (Fig. 17.VIII.1).
- The marked incision line is infiltrated with tumescent solution to provide analgesia.
- The incision is made through the skin and subcutaneous tissues. When this is done, the fascia lata will be exposed as a shiny white layer and will feel thick.
- The anterior and posterior skin flaps are raised superficial to the fascia lata for about 4 cm in either direction, to expose the fascia lata for harvest.
- The fascia lata is now ready for harvest. Usually, a width of about 4 cm and a length according to requirement is harvested. The required dimensions of the fascia lata is marked and incised all around with no. 15 blade. The harvested graft is placed in normal saline solution.
- If it is possible, the defect in the fascia lata is repaired with 3.0 polypropylene continuous sutures. If it is not possible, the defect is left as such and the wound is closed in layers: subcutaneous tissues with 3.0 vicryl, and skin with 3.0 polypropylenes subcuticular sutures.
- Sterile dressings and elastocrepe compression bandage is applied.

SECTION

18

Proformas

Microsurgery Recording Chart

Name: Date:
Age: Sex: P. S. Number:
Diagnosis:
Procedure:

Step	*Time of starting*	*Time of completing*
Anesthesia: Team:		
Recipient site: Team:		
Donor site: Team:		
Time of division of pedicle		
Vein 1: Vessels anastomosed: Team: Suture material used:		
Artery: Vessels anastomosed: Team: Suture material used:		
Vein 2: Vessels anastomosed: Team: Suture material used:		
Other: Vessels anastomosed: Team: Suture material used:		
Other: Vessels anastomosed: Team: Suture material used:		
Time of release of clamps		
Warm ischemia time		

Brachial Plexus Injury Evaluation

II

P.S. Number: Date:

Name: Age/Sex:

Side involved:

Date of accident:

Duration since injury:

Mode of injury: Road traffic accidents (RTA)/Industrial/Fall from height/Birth

Nature of injury: Low energy/High energy

Mechanism of injury: Neck shoulder separation/arm shoulder separation

History of pain: Continuous/occasional/No pain

Other injuries: Head/spine/clavicle/lower limb

Shift of head away from injured side: Yes/No

Horner's syndrome: Yes/No

Dislocation of shoulder: Yes/No

Swelling in supraclavicular region: Yes/No

Tinel's sign at supraclavicular region: Yes/No

Peripheral pulses:

Muscles/groups tested	*Muscle power grading (M0–M5)*
Trapezius	
Rhomboids	
Serratus anterior	
Shoulder abduction	
Shoulder adduction	
Shoulder flexion	
Shoulder extension	
Shoulder external rotation	
Shoulder internal rotation	
Elbow flexion	
Elbow extension	

Investigation reports and findings:
X-ray cervical spine:
X-ray chest—in inspiration and in expiration:
X-ray shoulder:
Computed tomography (CT) myelography:
Magnetic resonance imaging (MRI) scan:
Electromyography (EMG) studies:
Probable level of lesion:
Probable site of lesion:
Probable nature of lesion:

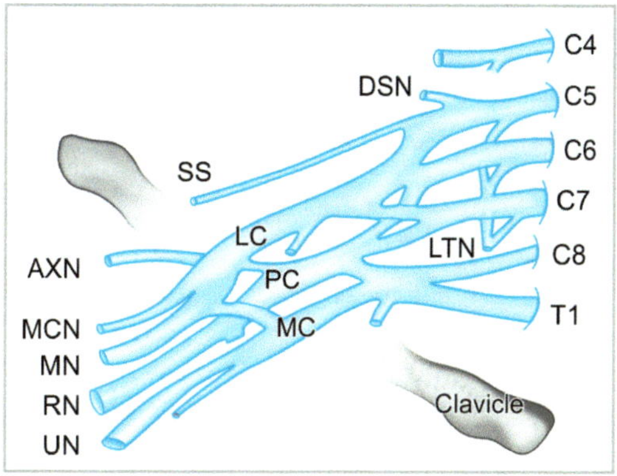

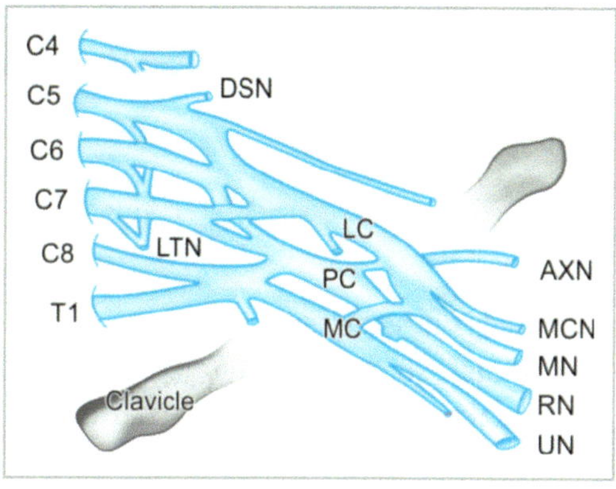

Plan:

Contracture of Upper Limb

Proforma for Assessment of Contracture on Upper Limb

P.S. Number: Date:
Name: Age/Sex:
Side involved:
Part involved:
Associated contractures:
Longitudinal extent of the contracture:
Quality of the skin over the contracted segment:
If scar is present, nature of scar:
Presence of ulcers, sinuses on the contracted segment:
Attitude of the upper limb/hand:
Position of the joints:

	Metacarpophalangeal (MCP) joint	*Proximal interphalangeal (PIP) joint*	*Distal interphalangeal (DIP) joint*
Index finger			
Middle finger			
Ring finger			
Little finger			
Thumb			

	Position
Wrist	
Elbow	
Axilla	

Range of motion at the joints:

	MCP joint		*PIP joint*		*DIP joint*	
	Active	***Passive***	***Active***	***Passive***	***Active***	***Passive***
Index finger						
Middle finger						
Ring finger						
Little finger						
Thumb						

	Flexion	*Extension*
Wrist		
Elbow		
Axilla		

Involvement of finger web spaces:
Involvement of nail complexes:
Involvement of thumb web:
Size of apparent defect:
Size of true defect:
Plan:

Dupuytren's Contracture Evaluation

IV

Evaluated by:

P.S. Number: Date:

Name: Age/Sex:

Side involved:

Date of accident:

Duration since injury:

Cause of injury:

History of: Diabetes mellitus/alcohol intake/epilepsy

Family history: Yes/No

Symptoms: Tightness in the palm/Nodules/Contracture of the fingers/Maceration of skin

Nodules: Number and site

Palpable cords:

Extent:

Position of the joints:

Contracture on the fingers	*MCP joint (a)*	*PIP joint (b)*	*DIP joint (c)*	*Total (a + b + c)*	*Stage*
Index finger					
Middle finger					
Ring finger					
Little finger					
Thumb					

Plan:

Volkmann's Ischemic Contracture Evaluation

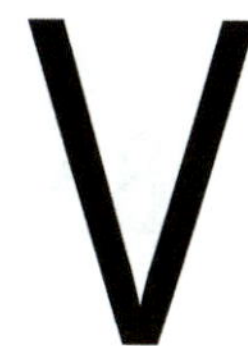

Evaluated by:
P.S. Number: Date:
Name: Age/Sex:
Side involved:
Date of accident:
Duration since injury:
Nature of injury:

Criteria to assess	*Type I*	*Type II*	*Type III*
Skin	Supple	Scarred	Contracture
Intrinsic muscles	Normal	Palsy	Contracture
Peripheral pulses	Present	+/–	+/–
Position of wrist	Normal	Flexion	Flexion contracture
Position of forearm	Normal	Fixed in pronation	Fixed in pronation
Position of thumb	Normal	Simian thumb	Adduction contracture
Position of fingers	Flexion	Claw	Intrinsic plus
Sensation	Normal	Loss of sensation	Loss
Finger flexion	Volkmann's sign	Weak flexion	Contracture
Fingers affected	Not all fingers	All the fingers	All the fingers
Joints	Supple	Stiff	Stiff
Power of flexion of fingers	Good	Weak	Contracture
Power of flexion of thumb	Good	Weak	Contracture
Extension of fingers	Present	+/–	+/–

Plan:

Sequence of plan:

Bone Problem Evaluation

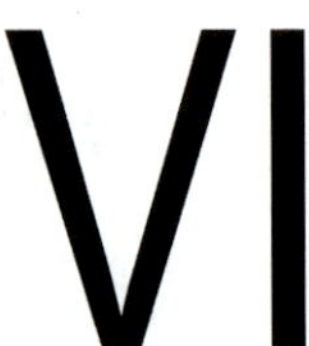

Evaluated by:

P.S. Number: Date:

Name: Age/Sex:

Side involved:

Date of accident:

Duration since injury:

Cause of injury:

Position of the joints of the fingers:

	MCP joint	*PIP joint*	*DIP joint*
Index finger			
Middle finger			
Ring finger			
Little finger			

Position of the joints of the thumb:

CMC joint	*MCP joint*	*IP joint*

Range of movements of the joints:

	MCP joint		*PIP joint*		*DIP joint*	
	Active	*Passive*	*Active*	*Passive*	*Active*	*Passive*
Index finger						
Middle finger						
Ring finger						
Little finger						
			IP joint			
			Active	*Passive*		
Thumb						

X-ray findings:
Malunion:
Nonunion:
Infection:
Sinus/scar:
Level of deformity:
Associated injuries:

Joint Problem Evaluation

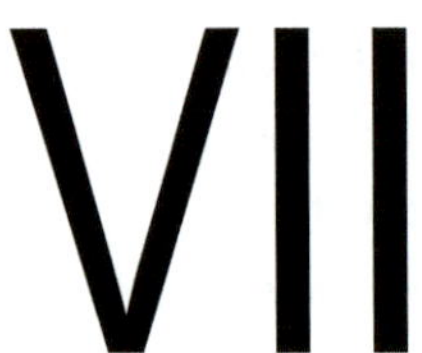

Evaluated by:
P.S. Number: Date:
Name: Age/Sex:
Side involved:
Date of accident:
Duration since injury:
Cause of injury:
Local symptoms: Pain/Swelling

Constitutional symptoms: Fever/malaise:

Position of the joints of the fingers:

	MCP joint	*PIP joint*	*DIP joint*
Index finger			
Middle finger			
Ring finger			
Little finger			

Position of the joints of the thumb:

Carpometacarpal (CMC) joint	*MCP joint*	*Interphalangeal (IP) joint*

Range of movements of the joints:

	MCP joint		PIP joint		DIP joint	
	Active	Passive	Active	Passive	Active	Passive
Index finger						
Middle finger						
Ring finger						
Little finger						
			IP joint			
			Active	Passive		
Thumb						

X-ray findings:
Nature of articular surfaces:
Congruity of articular spaces:
Joint space:
Status of bones proximal and distal to the joint:
Plan:

Tendon Injury Evaluation

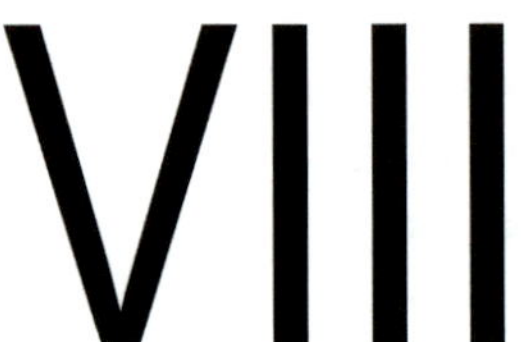

Evaluated by:
P.S. Number: Date:
Name: Age/Sex:
Side involved:
Date of accident:
Duration since injury: Less than 10 days/10 days–3 months/3 months–1 year/greater than 1 year
Nature of injury: Blunt/penetrating/assault/industrial/avulsion
Nature of scar: Soft and supple/indurated/hypertrophic/contracture
Fingers involved:
Tendons involved:
Sensation on the tips of fingers:
Associated fractures: No/united well/malunion/nonunion
Range of motion in the joints:

	MCP joint		*PIP joint*		*DIP joint*	
	Active	*Passive*	*Active*	*Passive*	*Active*	*Passive*
Index finger						
Middle finger						
Ring finger						
Little finger						
Thumb						

Plan:
Physiotherapy evaluation:

Index

Page numbers followed by *f* refer to figure and *t* refer to table, respectively.

L

M

N

O

W

Z